Long QT Syndrome

Guest Editor

SILVIA G. PRIORI, MD, PhD

CARDIAC ELECTROPHYSIOLOGY CLINICS

www.cardiacEP.theclinics.com

Consulting Editors
RANJAN K. THAKUR, MD, MPH, MBA, FHRS
ANDREA NATALE, MD, FACC, FHRS

March 2012 • Volume 4 • Number 1

SAUNDERS an imprint of ELSEVIER, Inc.

W.B. SAUNDERS COMPANY
A Division of Elsevier Inc.

1600 John F. Kennedy Boulevard • Suite 1800 • Philadelphia, Pennsylvania 19103-2899

http://www.theclinics.com

CARDIAC ELECTROPHYSIOLOGY CLINICS Volume 4, Number 1
March 2012 ISSN 1877-9182, ISBN-13: 978-1-4557-3835-9

Editor: Barbara Cohen-Kligerman
Developmental Editor: Teia Stone

Cardiac Electrophysiology Clinics (ISSN 1877-9182) is published quarterly by Elsevier Inc., 360 Park Avenue South, New York, NY 10010-1710. Months of issue are March, June, September, and December. Subscription prices are $180.00 per year for US individuals, $266.00 per year for US institutions, $95.00 per year for US students and residents, $202.00 per year for Canadian individuals, $297.00 per year for Canadian institutions, $258.00 per year for international individuals, $318.00 per year for international institutions and $136.00 per year for Canadian and foreign students/residents. To receive student/resident rate, orders must be accompanied by name of affilliated institution, date of term, and the signature of program/residency coordinator on institution letterhead. Orders will be billed at individual rate until proof of status is received. Foreign air speed delivery is included in all Clinics subscription prices. All prices are subject to change without notice. **POSTMASTER:** Send address changes to Cardiac Electrophysiology Clinics, Elsevier Health Sciences Division, Subscription Customer Service, 3251 Riverport Lane, Maryland Heights, MO 63043. **Customer Service: 1-800-654-2452 (US and Canada). From outside of the US and Canada, call 314-477-8871. Fax: 314-447-8029. E-mail: JournalsCustomerService-usa@elsevier.com (for print support); JournalsOnlineSupport-usa@elsevier.com (for online support).**

Reprints. For copies of 100 or more of articles in this publication, please contact the Commercial Reprints Department, Elsevier Inc., 360 Park Avenue South, New York, NY 10010-1710. Tel.: 212-633-3812; Fax: 212-462-1935; E-mail: reprints@elsevier.com.

Printed and bound by CPI Group (UK) Ltd, Croydon, CR0 4YY

Transferred to Digital Print 2012

Differential temporal change of the heart rate corrected QT Interval (QTc) to epinephrine provocative testing in LQT1, 2, and 3 patients (Shimizu Protocol). See "Diagnostic Evaluation of Long QT Syndrome" by Wataru Shimizu, MD, PhD, for further details.

Contributors

CONSULTING EDITORS

RANJAN K. THAKUR, MD, MPH, MBA, FHRS
Professor of Medicine, and Director,
Arrhythmia Service, Thoracic and
Cardiovascular Institute, Sparrow Health
System, Michigan State University,
Lansing, Michigan

ANDREA NATALE, MD, FACC, FHRS
Executive Medical Director of the Texas
Cardiac Arrhythmia Institute at St David's
Medical Center, Austin, Texas; Consulting
Professor, Division of Cardiology, Stanford
University, Palo Alto, California; Clinical
Associate Professor of Medicine, Case
Western Reserve University, Cleveland, Ohio;
Senior Clinical Director, EP Services, California
Pacific Medical Center, San Francisco,
California; Department of Biomedical
Engineering, University of Texas, Austin, Texas

GUEST EDITOR

SILVIA G. PRIORI, MD, PhD
Director of Molecular Cardiology, Division
of Molecular Cardiology, IRCCS Fondazione
Salvatore Maugeri; Department of Molecular
Medicine, University of Pavia, Pavia, Italy;
Cardiovascular Genetics Program, Leon H.
Charney Division of Cardiology, NYU Langone
Medical Center, New York, New York

AUTHORS

CHARLES ANTZELEVITCH, PhD
Gordon K. Moe Scholar, Executive Director
and Director of Research, Masonic Medical
Research Laboratory, Utica, New York

ANDREW D. BLAUFOX, MD, FACC, FHRS
Section Chief, Electrophysiology, Division of
Pediatric Cardiology, Department of
Pediatrics, The Heart Center, The Steven and
Alexandra Cohen Children's Medical Center of
New York; Associate Professor of Pediatrics,
North Shore – LIJ Hofstra School of Medicine,
New Hyde Park, New York

RAFFAELLA BLOISE, MD
Molecular Cardiology, IRCCS Fondazione
Salvatore Maugeri; Department of Molecular
Medicine, University of Pavia, Pavia, Italy

ILAN GOLDENBERG, MD
Heart Research Follow-up Program,
Cardiology Division, University of
Rochester Medical Center, Rochester,
New York

ELIZABETH S. KAUFMAN, MD
Professor of Medicine, MetroHealth Campus
of Case Western Reserve University, Heart
and Vascular Research Center, MetroHealth
Medical Center, Cleveland, Ohio

ANDREA MAZZANTI, MD
Instituto de Investigación Biomédica de la
Universidad de A Coruña (INIBIC), Instituto
de Ciencias de la Salud, A Coruña, Spain

ARTHUR J. MOSS, MD
Heart Research Follow-up Program, Cardiology Division, University of Rochester Medical Center, Rochester, New York

CARLO NAPOLITANO, MD, PhD
Division of Molecular Cardiology, Fondazione Salvatore Maugeri, Via Salvatore Maugeri, Pavia, Italy

SILVIA G. PRIORI, MD, PhD
Director of Molecular Cardiology, Division of Molecular Cardiology, IRCCS Fondazione Salvatore Maugeri; Department of Molecular Medicine, University of Pavia, Pavia, Italy; Cardiovascular Genetics Program, Leon H. Charney Division of Cardiology, NYU Langone Medical Center, New York, New York

ERIC SCHULZE-BAHR, MD
Professor, Director of the Institute for Genetics of Heart Diseases, Department of Cardiology and Angiology, University Hospital Münster, Münster, Germany

PETER J. SCHWARTZ, MD, FACC, FAHA, FESC, FHRS
Professor and Chairman of Cardiology, Department of Molecular Medicine, University of Pavia; Department of Cardiology, Fondazione IRCCS Policlinico S. Matteo, Pavia, Italy; Cardiovascular Genetics

Laboratory, Department of Medicine, Hatter Institute for Cardiovascular Research in Africa, The Cape Heart Centre, University of Cape Town; Department of Medicine, University of Stellenbosch, Cape Town, South Africa; Chair of Sudden Death, Department of Family and Community Medicine, College of Medicine, King Saud University, Riyadh, Kingdom of Saudi Arabia

WATARU SHIMIZU, MD, PhD
Division of Arrhythmia and Electrophysiology, Department of Cardiovascular Medicine, National Cerebral and Cardiovascular Center, Suita, Osaka, Japan

SERGE SICOURI, MD
Research Scientist, Experimental Cardiology, Masonic Medical Research Laboratory, Utica, New York

WOJCIECH ZAREBA, MD, PhD
Heart Research Follow-up Program, Cardiology Division, University of Rochester Medical Center, Rochester, New York

OHAD ZIV, MD
Assistant Professor of Medicine, Case Western Reserve University, Heart and Vascular Research Center, MetroHealth Medical Center, Cleveland, Ohio

Contents

Genetic investigations have identified many inherited arrhythmia syndromes without the presence of structural heart disease. Congenital long QT syndrome (LQTS) is a paradigm for this because it is the first, and genetically mostly dissected, familial arrhythmia syndrome. The prevalence of prolonged QT interval durations in the first 3 decades is estimated at between 1:2,000 and 1:3,000 (0.05%–0.033%). At least 13 LQTS genes define distinct genetic subforms, some of which are quite rare and associated with extra-cardiac manifestations. More than 700 mutations have been documented, and they are randomly distributed within the coding regions of the LQTS genes.

Prolongation of the QT interval is caused by an increase in the duration of action potential (APD) of ventricular myocytes. It can result from several causes, including congenital defects, or can occur in response to an increasing number and diversity of drugs that prolong APD. Accentuation of spatial dispersion of refractoriness within the ventricular myocardium, secondary to exaggerated transmural or transseptal dispersion of repolarization, is the principal arrhythmogenic substrate in acquired and congenital long QT syndrome (LQTS). This article discusses the molecular, genetic, cellular, and ionic mechanisms underlying the development of arrhythmogenesis associated with LQTS.

Congenital long QT syndrome (LQTS) is one of the heritable channelopathies characterized by prolongation of QT interval. An estimated 30% to 40% of genetically affected subjects have concealed LQTS with a normal or borderline rate-corrected QT interval at rest in congenital LQTS. The genetic subtypes LQTS, LQT1, LQT2, and LQT3 comprise the vast majority of genotyped LQTS and approximately 75% of all LQTS. In this article, the role of provocative testing in the evaluation of congenital LQTS, specifically diagnosing (unmasking) concealed LQTS and predicting genotypes of LQTS (LQT1, LQT2, and LQT3), is reviewed.

This article reviews the manner in which age and gender affect electrocardiographic measurements of repolarization and therefore the QT interval. The authors detail the effects of age and gender on clinical outcomes in long QT syndrome and review how these modulations drive treatment recommendations. They also discuss basic research that has recently begun to shed light on these clinical phenomena and may give insight into potential future treatments.

The long QT syndrome is one of the most prevalent and studied among the inherited arrhythmogenic conditions that expose individuals to a high risk of sudden death, from early infancy throughout the entire lifespan. The hallmark of the syndrome is its heterogeneity in genetic background, phenotypic manifestations, responses to therapy, and prognosis. ß-Blockers are successful in protecting most patients from adverse events, but some remain vulnerable despite antiadrenergic drugs, and require more aggressive therapeutic approaches. Effective stratification based on clinical and genetic parameters is crucial to identify patients with the highest risk and to avoid overtreatment.

There are few data concerning long QT syndrome (LQTS) in fetuses, neonates, and infants. Although most patients with LQTS do not have significant symptoms at this age, those who present with severe symptoms in early life have a worse prognosis. Early recognition of these symptoms as manifestations of LQTS and institution of appropriate therapy may prevent sudden cardiac death and SIDS in these children. Unfortunately, traditional medical therapy may not be effective in the most at-risk children and more aggressive management is needed; however, because of the size of these children, innovative approaches to providing this therapy are needed.

This article reviews the role of the sympathetic nervous system in long QT syndrome (LQTS), in light of clinical and personal experience. The evolution of concepts related to LQTS is examined after 40 years of research and treatment. Studies stimulated by the sympathetic imbalance hypothesis have generated many unsuspected novel data and have provided an extremely strong rationale for the therapeutic use of left cardiac sympathetic denervation to prevent ventricular fibrillation, not only in LQTS but also in other life-threatening diseases associated with high risk for arrhythmic sudden death.

The implanted cardioverter-defibrillator (ICD) is frequently used in the management of high-risk patients with long QT syndrome (LQTS). The following factors indicate a high risk for aborted cardiac arrest or death: corrected QT interval prolongation, history of aborted cardiac arrest (ACA), history of syncope, and information on mutations. History of ACA or syncope despite ß-blocker treatment is an approved ICD indication in patients with LQTS. Programming of ICDs requires further investigation because there is no uniform protocol to decrease the risk of therapies delivered when self-terminating episodes of torsade de pointes ventricular tachycardia might occur.

How to Interpret Results of Genetic Testing and Counsel Families   97

Raffaella Bloise and Silvia G. Priori

The human genome project has facilitated the identification of disease-causing genes and has promoted the introduction of DNA screening in clinical medicine. The application of molecular diagnostics to patient management has generated the need to design novel models of care for patients with inherited diseases. A specific educational track to train arrhythmologists in clinical electrophysiology is needed. This article discusses the complexity of the interpretation of genetic testing in long QT syndrome. The challenges that are present in the interpretation of genetic results and the tools that may overcome the hurdle posed by unknown DNA variants are also discussed.

Cardiac Electrophysiology Clinics

THE CLINICS ARE AVAILABLE ONLINE!

Access your subscription at:
www.theclinics.com

Foreword
The "Goldilocks Principle": QT Interval—"Not Too Long, Not Too Short, Just Right"

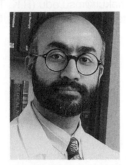
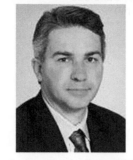

Ranjan K. Thakur, MD, MPH, MBA, FHRS   Andrea Natale, MD, FHRS
Consulting Editors

The "Goldilocks principle," derived from a children's story, *Goldilocks and the Three Bears*, states that an observed phenomenon must fall within a certain range, as opposed to reaching extremes, reflecting the principle of equilibrium. It has been described in biology, economics, engineering, astrophysics, medicine and other fields. The principle certainly seems to apply to the QT interval and augurs problems if the QT interval is too short or too long. The focus of this issue of *Cardiac Electrophysiology Clinics* is on the long QT syndrome (LQTS).

While the first case of LQTS was described by Meissner over 150 years ago, little was known about it until relatively recently. In our lifetime we have seen the evolution of our understanding develop from a cursory phenotypic description to a much more nuanced understanding of clinical syndromes, risk stratification, genetics, molecular mechanisms, and therapies. This was only possible because of an international effort: establishment of the International Long QT Registry by Crampton, Moss, and Schwartz in 1979, a worldwide effort to understand the variegated clinical presentations, an internationally accepted nomenclature for classification, efforts on the genetic, molecular and therapeutic fronts.

Sudden death and familial occurrence were described in the first reported case by Meissner. It has become clear that sudden death is arrhythmic in nature. In fact, it was the risk of sudden death that led to such intense international interest in this entity. Now, we also understand the genes involved and how they cause molecular perturbations that predispose to arrhythmias. We can screen for these genes in suspected cases or the proband's family members and, thus, can risk-stratify and treat these patients more appropriately.

Dr Silvia Priori has been at the forefront in deepening our understanding of LQTS. We were delighted when she accepted our invitation to assemble a panel of international experts to summarize the present understanding of this syndrome for the busy electrophysiologist who must deal with clinical decisions.

The reader will find articles ranging from the level of the laboratory bench to the bedside. For example, Dr Antzelevitch describes mechanisms underlying arrhythmogenesis; Dr Shimizu discusses diagnostic evaluation, and Dr Priori expounds on risk stratification. Dr Moss discusses the role of the implantable cardioverter defibrillator for prevention of sudden cardiac death in these patients, and Dr Priori also discusses how to interpret the results of genetic testing in these probands and their families and how to counsel them.

We congratulate Dr Priori and her panel of experts for their review articles and expect that

Card Electrophysiol Clin 4 (2012) ix–x
doi:10.1016/j.ccep.2012.01.005
1877-9182/12/$ – see front matter © 2012 Elsevier Inc. All rights reserved.

readers will find this issue useful in clinical practice.

Ranjan K. Thakur, MD, MPH, MBA, FHRS
Arrhythmia Service
E.W. Sparrow Thoracic and Cardiovascular Institute
Michigan State University
1200 East Michigan Avenue, Suite 580
Lansing, MI 48912, USA

Andrea Natale, MD, FHRS
Texas Cardiac Arrhythmia Institute
Center for Atrial Fibrillation at
St. David's Medical Center
1015 East 32nd Street, Suite 516
Austin, TX 78705, USA

E-mail addresses:
thakur@msu.edu (R.K. Thakur)
andrea.natale@stdavids.com (A. Natale)

Preface

Long QT Syndrome: From Epidemiology to Molecular Genetics—The Disease that has Opened a New Chapter in Electrophysiology

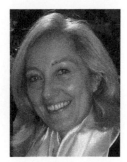

Silvia G. Priori, MD, PhD
Guest Editor

Since its early description by the Italian physician Romano[1] and the Irish doctor Ward,[2] long QT syndrome (LQTS) has attracted the interest of the pediatric as well as the cardiologic community for its peculiar electrocardiographic manifestations and high lethality.

The clinical contribution of the pivotal work of Drs Moss and Schwartz in the 1970s led to the identification of the therapeutic value of left cardiac denervation[3] and to the definition of diagnostic criteria.[4] Over the years our understanding of the disease has advanced thanks to the establishment of an International Registry initiated by Drs Moss, Schwartz, and Crampton in the 1980s. The turning point for LQTS was, however, represented by the discovery of its genetic basis by Mark Keating and his group in the mid-1990s.[5–7] With the introduction of molecular genetics, the diagnosis and management of the syndrome have been rewritten, incorporating data from genotype-phenotype correlation studies that have revealed the complexity and heterogeneity of the disease.

Based on the unique profile of LQTS and its historical value as the disease that has paved the way to the development of molecular arrhythmology, it is virtually impossible to recapitulate the broad knowledge gathered in the field in a single article. For this reason we have called for the expertise and the vision of physicians who have made prominent contributions to LQTS to develop this review effort.

This volume summarizes the clinical features of the disease and its management strategies as they appear now, almost 50 years after its description by Dr Romano, a graduate of the University of Pavia, where Dr Schwartz and I work and have the honor to continue to study the LQTS.

I wish to thank all the authors for the effort of writing original and updated articles with the intent to disseminate knowledge on the management of the disease to the benefit of the affected families worldwide.

Silvia G. Priori, MD, PhD
Molecular Cardiology
IRCCS Fondazione Salvatore Maugeri
Pavia, Italy
Department of Molecular Medicine
University of Pavia
Pavia, Italy
Cardiovascular Genetics Program
Leon H. Charney Division of Cardiology
NYU Langone Medical Center
New York, NY, USA

E-mail address:
silvia.priori@nyumc.org

Card Electrophysiol Clin 4 (2012) xi–xii
doi:10.1016/j.ccep.2012.01.004
1877-9182/12/$ – see front matter © 2012 Elsevier Inc. All rights reserved.

cardiacEP.theclinics.com

REFERENCES

1. Romano C, Gemme G, Pongiglione R. Aritmie cardiache rare dell'età pediatrica. Clin Pediatr (Phila) 1963; 45:656–83.
2. Ward OC. A new familial cardiac syndrome in children. J Ir Med Assoc 1964;54:103–6.
3. Moss AJ, McDonald J. Unilateral cervicothoracic sympathetic ganglionectomy for the treatment of long QT interval syndrome. N Engl J Med 1971;285:903–4.
4. Schwartz PJ, Moss AJ, Vincent GM, et al. Diagnostic criteria for the long QT syndrome: an update. Circulation 1993;88:782–4.
5. Wang Q, Shen J, Splawski I, et al. SCN5A mutations associated with an inherited cardiac arrhythmia, long QT syndrome. Cell 1995;80:805–11.
6. Curran ME, Splawski I, Timothy KW, et al. A molecular basis for cardiac arrhythmia: HERG mutations cause long QT syndrome. Cell. 1995;80:795–803.
7. Wang Q, Curran ME, Splawski I, et al. Positional cloning of a novel potassium channel gene: KVLQT1 mutations cause cardiac arrhythmias. Nat Genet 1996;12:17–23.

Long QT Syndromes: Genetic Basis

Eric Schulze-Bahr, MD[a,b,c],*

KEYWORDS

- Long QT syndrome • Ion channel • Repolarization • Gene

In the last two decades, genetic investigations have identified many inherited arrhythmia syndromes without the presence of structural heart disease (so-called primary electrical heart diseases). Congenital long QT syndrome (LQTS) is a paradigm for this because it is the first and genetically mostly dissected, familial arrhythmia syndrome. The prevalence of prolonged QT interval durations (the clinical hallmark of LQTS) is estimated at between 1:2,000 and 1:3,000 (0.05%–0.033%).[1–4] To date, at least 13 LQTS genes (LQT-1 to LQT-13, mostly encoding cardiac ion channel protein components; **Table 1**) define distinct subforms. Autosomal dominant as well as recessive and de novo forms of LQTS are known. More than 700 mutations have been published, and they are randomly distributed within the coding regions of the LQTS genes. Gene-specific and Web-based mutation databases mean while exist and allow identification of LQTS mutations in other publications. **Box 1** lists a few examples of such databases.

In most cases, each mutation represents a single (family-specific, private) rather than common (hot spot) event. Founder mutations in LQTS genes as a common disease cause only occur in some populations with a confounding substructure (mainly LQT-1).[5–9]

Compound or digenic heterozygosity (ie, 2 mutations in a patient with LQTS, either on different alleles or genes) causing a more severe phenotype

can be observed in 5% to 10% of patients with LQTS[10–13] and should be considered in the presence of severe QT prolongation or discordance of the clinical phenotype and genotype in a family with LQTS. Interpreting the significance of a genetic test result in the context of insufficient clinical data and/or disease evidence is challenging for physicians; apart from nonsynonymous LQTS gene mutations, there is a widespread natural (polymorphic) variance in amino acids that often has ethnic-specific differences in allele frequencies.[14,15] The cardiac sodium channel gene SCN5A, identified as the cause for congenital LQT-3,[16] but also for Brugada syndrome, atrial and ventricular conduction diseases, sinus node dysfunction, and dilated cardiomyopathy, is such an example. In addition to heterogeneity with sometimes overlapping phenotypes,[17,18] many nonsynonymous amino acid exchanges are described that have subtle or potentially no in vitro effects on native sodium channel function.[19–28] In a recent study,[29] the frequency and localization of LQT-1 to LQT-3 mutations in cases and healthy controls (n>1,300) were compared. Gene variants were significantly more common in LQTS cases than in controls in each of the 3 genes, but to different degrees (0.29/LQTS vs 0.01/control; LQT-2, 0.28 vs 0.02; and LQT-3, 0.07 vs 0.03) with lower mutation rates among white LQTS cases and controls than among non-white individuals. On the localization within the 3 ion channel proteins, predicted estimated

This work was supported by the Leducq Foundation, Paris, France, and by the German Research Foundation, Bonn, Germany (DFG Schu1082/4-1 and Schu1082/4-2, DFG Ki653/13-1, SFB 656-C1) and by the IZKF (Schu01-012-11).

[a] Department of Cardiology and Angiology, Institute for Genetics of Heart Diseases, University Hospital Münster, Münster, Germany
[b] Interdisciplinary Center for Clinical Research (IZKF), Münster, Germany
[c] Collaborative Research Centre on Molecular Cardiovascular Imaging (SFB656) at the University of Münster, Münster, Germany
* Institut für Genetik von Herzerkrankungen (IfGH), Albert-Schweitzer-Campus 1 (Gebäude D3), Universitätsklinikum Münster, D-48145 Münster, Germany.
E-mail address: Eric.Schulze-Bahr@ukmuenster.de

Card Electrophysiol Clin 4 (2012) 1–16
doi:10.1016/j.ccep.2012.01.001

Table 1
LQTS: genes and dysfunction

Type	Gene	Chromosome	Protein	Dysfunction
LQTS, common subforms (>1%)				
LQT-1	KCNQ1	11p15.5	Kv7.1	I_{Ks} α-subunit, loss of function
LQT-2	KCNH2	7q35–q36	Kv11.1	I_{Kr} α-subunit, loss of function
LQT-3	SCN5A	3p21	Nav1.5	I_{Na} α-subunit, gain of function
LQTS, uncommon subforms (<1%)				
LQT-4	ANK2	4q25–q27	Ankyrin-B	Targeting/anchor protein, secondary loss of function (several target proteins)
LQT-5	KCNE1	21q22	MinK	I_{Ks} β-subunit, loss of function
?LQT-6	KCNE2	21q22	MiRP1	$?I_{Kr}$ β-subunit, loss of function
LQT-9	CAV3	3p25	Caveolin-3	Caveolae coat protein, secondary gain of function (Nav1.5)
LQT-10	SCN4B	11q23	Navb4	I_{Na} β-subunit, gain of function (Nav1.5)
LQT-11	AKAP9	7q21–q22	Yotiao	Adaptor molecule, loss of function (eg, Kv11.1)
LQT-12	SNTA1	20q11.2	α1-Syntrophin	Membrane scaffold, secondary gain of function (Nav1.5)
LQT-13	KCNJ5	11q24.3	Kir3.4/Girk4	$I_{K.ACh}$ α-subunit, loss of function
LQTS with extracardiac manifestations (rare)				
JLN-1 (JLNS; autosomal recessive)	KCNQ1	11p15.5	Kv7.1	I_{Ks} α-subunit, loss of function
JLN-2 (JLNS; autosomal recessive)	KCNE1	21q22	MinK	I_{Ks} β-subunit, loss of function
LQT-7 (ATS; autosomal dominant)	KCNJ2	17q24.3	Kir2.1	I_{K1} α-subunit, loss of function
LQT-8 (TS; autosomal dominant)	*CACNA1C*	12p13.3	Cav1.2	I_{LTCC} α-subunit, gain of function

Abbreviations: ATS, Andersen-Tawil syndrome; JLNS, Jervell and Lange-Nielsen syndrome; TS, Timothy syndrome.

probabilities for being a causative disease mutation were proposed.[29]

In 1993, the diagnostic criteria for LQTS were revised[30] because genetic information was not being used as part of the diagnostic procedure. Meanwhile, many publications describe how to standardize and measure electrocardiogram (ECG) parameters[31] and how to interpret QT correction formulas[32] to recognize QTc prolongation sufficiently. In our institution, LQTS is diagnosed by the presence of QTc prolongation together with at least 1 additional indicator, as shown in **Box 2**.

In a recent Heart Rhythm Society (HRS)/European Heart Rhythm Association (EHRA) expert consensus statement on genetic testing (**Box 3**),[33] genetic investigations in LQTS were clearly recommended (class I recommendation) in patients with a high suspicion for LQTS or in close family relatives of an index patient (proband) with a proven LQTS gene mutation. In addition, a stratified and rational genotyping approach starting with the common subforms (LQT-1 to LQT-3) has been recommended.[33] For rare LQTS forms with extracardiac manifestations, a direct sequencing approach of the causative genes (eg, LQT-7; see later discussion) may be appropriate.

Taken together, congenital LQTS is an example in which knowledge of the individual genetic information is followed by a triad of clinical

Box 1
Genetic mutation databases

http://www.fsm.it/cardmoc/

http://www.genomed.org/LOVD/introduction.html

http://www.hgmd.cf.ac.uk/docs/oth_mut.html

Box 2
Diagnosis of LQTS

1. QTc prolongation:

   a. At baseline or during higher heart rate (also provoked)

   b. Exclusion of secondary causes (eg, drugs or structural heart disease)

2. a. LQTS gene mutation

   and/or

   b. Familial LQTS

   and/or

   c. LQTS-related symptoms

Box 3
Genetic testing for LQTS, summary of expert consensus recommendations

Class I (recommended)

- Comprehensive or LQT-1 to LQT-3 (KCNQ1, KCNH2, and SCN5A) targeted LQTS genetic testing is recommended

  o For any patient in whom a cardiologist has established a strong clinical index of suspicion for LQTS

  o For any asymptomatic patient with QT prolongation defined as QTc greater than or equal to 480 milliseconds (prepuberty) or greater than or equal to 500 milliseconds (adults) in the absence of other clinical conditions

- Mutation-specific genetic testing is recommended for family members and other appropriate relatives following the identification of the LQTS-causative mutation in an index case

Class IIb (may be considered)

- Comprehensive or LQT-1 to LQT1-3 (*KCNQ1, KCNH2,* and *SCN5A*) targeted LQTS genetic testing may be considered

  o For any asymptomatic patient with otherwise idiopathic QTc values greater than or equal to 460 milliseconds (prepuberty) or greater than or equal to 480 milliseconds (adults)

Data from Ackerman MJ, Priori SG, Willems S, et al. HRS/EHRA expert consensus statement on the state of genetic testing for the channelopathies and cardiomyopathies this document was developed as a partnership between the Heart Rhythm Society (HRS) and the European Heart Rhythm Association (EHRA). Heart Rhythm 2011;8(8):1308–39.

consequences; for diagnostic purposes,[34] for therapeutic decisions[35] and lifestyle recommendations,[36–40] and probably for cardiac risk assessment.[41,42] These aspects are outside the scope of this article.

CONGENITAL LQTS
1. Common Genetic Subforms (>1%)

Mutations in the first 3 ion channel genes to be identified (LQT-1, LQT-2, LQT-3) are still the cornerstone for more than 70% of index cases for genotyping.[43–45] Typically, not all mutation carriers (only 70%–80%, author's own data) showed a prolonged QTc interval (>450–460 milliseconds) at baseline ECG and, in consequence, a significant number of mutation carriers showed a remarkable overlap with unaffected family members.[45] Incomplete penetrance of ECG manifestation (ie, QTc prolongation) was higher in LQT-1 and LQT-5 (I_{Ks} channel gene) mutation carriers.

In 1991, a genome-wide analysis first reported linkage of markers on human chromosome 11 with congenital LQTS[46]; 5 years later, in 1996, positional cloning methods established mutations in a potassium channel gene, *KCNQ1* (formerly KVLQT1; chromosome 11p15.5), as the cause for autosomal dominant LQTS (LQT-1).[8] The LQT-1 gene encodes the α-subunit of the slowly activating, delayed outward rectifying K+ channel (I_{Ks}) and is thought to have a tetrameric conformation with additional β-subunits (MinK; LQT-5) and other, regulatory proteins (see later discussion). The protein Kv7.1, encoded by KCNQ1, when coexpressed with MinK, yields potassium currents that activate slowly on depolarization, displays no inactivation, and deactivates slowly during repolarization. I_{Ks} is markedly enhanced by α-adrenergic stimulation; patients with LQT-1 gene mutations have a reduction in myocellular repolarization that becomes especially apparent at higher heart rates during emotional and/or physical activity.[40,47,48] LQT-1 is the most common type of autosomal dominant LQTS (~30%) and is caused by mutations resulting in a loss of function, either by reducing I_{Ks} channel density (eg, truncating or hypomorphic mutations) or through a dominant negative effect (eg, I_{Ks} suppression of wild-type function caused by mutation). More than 250 different LQT-1 mutations are known; most are missense (nonsynonymous) mutations. The multiple mechanisms by which I_{Ks} channel function is disturbed have only been investigated for some of these. The heterologous expression system and conditions for in vitro investigations have a strong influence on the mutant ion channels (eg, the LQT-1 A341V mutation).[8,49–51] As noted for other ion channel disorders, mutations in the *KCNQ1* gene may have overlapping clinical phenotypes (eg, with atrial fibrillation or sinus node dysfunction)[52–54] or, alternatively, a short QT syndrome (SQTS) when linked to a gain of function.[55] Imboden and colleagues[56] reported on the distribution of mutant alleles in families with 484 LQT-1 and 269 LQT-2 to investigate the known female predominance of affected family members. In the offspring of the female LQT-1 (and all LQT-2) carriers, classic mendelian inheritance ratios were not observed, and an increased maternal transmission of mutant LQTS alleles was observed, possibly contributing to the excess of female patients with autosomal dominant LQTS.[56]

In 1995, another potassium channel gene, hERG (human ether-a-go-go–related gene), now referred to as *KCNH2*, was identified as being responsible for LQT-2 (chromosome 7q35-q36) and is linked to drug-induced prolonged repolarization.[57,58] *KCNH2* encodes the α-subunit (Kv11.1) of the I_{Kr} potassium channel, which is activated on depolarization and rapidly inactivated thereafter, resulting in a small outward K+ current near the end of the action potential upstroke (phase III). However, during early repolarization, the channel rapidly recovers from inactivation to produce large I_{Kr} amplitudes and then closes (deactivates) slowly in a voltage-independent process. LQT-2 is the second most prevalent subtype of LQTS (25%–30%) and is caused by loss-of-function mutations. Similarly to LQT-1, and shown by the use of mammalian heterologous expression systems, most LQT-2 mutants are hypomorphic and result in a trafficking defect by moving mutant Kv11.1 proteins to the sarcolemma or immature proteins.[59–62] More than 300 LQT-2 mutations, mainly missense mutations, have been found so far. Homozygous mutations are an exception and result in a severe, early-onset phenotype.[63–66] A few gain-of-function mutations in KCNH2 are linked to SQT-1.[67–69]

Also in 1995, mutations in the *SCN5A* gene (chromosome 3p22.2) encoding the α-subunit of the cardiac isoform of the voltage-gated sodium channel (Nav1.5) were first described to cause LQT-3 (10%).[16,70] Of the 80 mutations known so far, all are missense or in-frame mutations, because a loss of function (eg, through a frameshift, splicing, or nonsense mutation) would result in reduced depolarization forces and in a different phenotype with a reduced conduction (eg, Brugada syndrome, atrial block, or standstill). Opening of the Nav1.5 channel allows a rapid membrane depolarization; the cardiac Nav1.5 channel is a multimeric protein complex that regulates its gating, cellular localization, intracellular transport, and degradation.

A gain of function and increase in I_{Na} is caused by either impaired inactivation., (ie, failure to inactivate completely) or an increase in the so-called window current. The latter is generally attributable to a shift of voltage dependence of steady-state inactivation toward more depolarized membrane potentials leaving an increased window of inward sodium current. Among the 15 *SCN5A* (LQT-3) missense mutations that have been characterized in heterologous expression systems so far, various mechanisms that are consistent with the hypothesis of an increased I_{Na} current being the cause for LQT-3 have been shown.[71,72] Some patients with typical *SCN5A* gain of function have suffered from atrial fibrillation alone or mixed phenotypes, most likely caused by the presence of unknown modifying factors or additional changes of Nav1.5 function by a reduction of I_{Na} current amplitude.[17,73–77] The observation that some *SCN5A* mutations harbor properties for different arrhythmogenic phenotypes suggested the clinical administration of sodium channel blockers (eg, mexiletine) to patients with LQT-3.[78–81] Drug response and also the clinical expressivity of *SCN5A* mutation carriers have been proposed to depend on the additional presence of *SCN5A* polymorphisms. One example is the S1103Y variant that is predominantly present in 13% of African Americans and is associated with accelerated channel activation.[28] For other variants, such as H558R[82–85] or the splice variant 1077delQ,[21,25,86] the overall role of *SCN5A* polymorphisms in disease modulation is not yet conclusive.

2. Uncommon or Rare Genetic Subforms (<1%)

In patients with congenital LQTS and absence of extracardiac features, several rare subforms (n = 9: LQT-4,5, LQT-6, LQT-9–13) exist that each has a relative LQTS mutation frequency of less than 1%. Except for the genes for the subform LQT-4 (*ANKB* or *ANK2*; ankyrin-B)[87,88] and LQT-13 (*KCNJ5*),[89] which have been found through genome-wide genetic linkage, all others have been identified using candidate gene approaches.

Rare Potassium Channel–Related Subforms

The LQT-5 gene, *KCNE1* on chromosome 21q22, encodes a small, auxiliary β-subunit (129 amino acids) called minimal potassium ion channel protein (MinK), which coassembles with 4 α-subunits (KCNQ1/K_VLQT1; LQT-1) to form functional delayed rectifier I_{Ks} potassium channels.[90,91] After the discovery that heterozygous loss-of-function mutations in the *KCNQ1* gene are linked to congenital repolarization abnormalities, it was shown that heterozygous mutations in KCNE1 also cause congenital LQTS.[92–98] The clinical phenotype is often mild and might, in the presence of only a slight QT prolongation and normal T-waves, be overlooked.[93,96] However, a series of recent investigations elucidated the functional importance of MinK in I_{Ks} channel function and regulation.[99] Nearly all *KCNE1* mutations are missense (nonsynonymous) mutations and result from loss of function in a reduction of I_{Ks} density and/or from altered biophysical properties. Recent investigations showed that defective I_{Ks} channel complex assembly,[100–103] intracellular subunit/channel trafficking,[104–106] or impaired channel regulation (eg, PIP_2 binding)[95,107,108] are consequences of altered MinK subunits.

G protein–activated inward rectifier potassium channels of type 1 and 4 (Girk1 and Girk4) form heteromeric complexes in cardiac and other tissues that exhibit all essential features of native cardiac acetylcholine (ACh)-dependent potassium ($I_{K,ACh}$) channels.[109] The *KCNJ5* gene, located on chromosome 11q24.3, has been linked to congenital LQTS in a single Chinese family,[89] but is also probably involved in atrial fibrillation (single patient)[110] and forms of hyperaldosteronism and/or aldosterone-producing adrenal adenomas as a somatic mosaic.[111] In the LQT-13 subform, affected members of a large, 4-generation Chinese family with autosomal dominant LQTS were carriers for a heterozygous G387R substitution at a highly conserved residue. In HEK293 cells co-transfected with Kir3.1/Girk1 (KCNJ3), a loss of function caused by the mutant Kir3.4/Girk4 was shown by a reduction of the $I_{K, ACh}$ inward potassium currents and reduced plasma membrane and intracellular Girk1/Girk4 protein levels.[89]

The *AKAP9* gene (yotiao; A-kinase anchor protein) located on chromosome 7q21.1 is responsible for another rare LQTS subform (LQT-11). Currently, only a single familial report exists, together with a growing set of functional data.[112] A-kinase anchor proteins have a critical role in excitable cell signaling; in the heart, AKAP9-associated protein kinase A (PKA) activity has been shown to modulate 3 important ion channel complexes including the I_{Ks} channel (LQT-1, LQT-5), the cardiac ryanodine receptor (RyR2; CPVT-1), and the L-type calcium channel (LQT-8). AKAP9/yotiao directly associates with Kv7.1/I_{Ks} channels and regulates their activity by PKA-dependent phosphorylation and gating.[99,113] The observation of a particular LQT-1 mutation (G589D) that interfered with the association of KCNQ1 with AKAP9/yotiao and I_{Ks} channel sensitivity to β-adrenergic stimulation[99] raised the

question of whether *AKAP9* gene mutations may alter the I_{Ks} channel activity. To date, this hypothesis has been proved in the rare identification of a heterozygous *AKAP9* mutation (S1570L) in an LQTS proband.[112] The mutant residue (S1570) is located close to the C-terminal binding site (1574–1643) for KCNQ1; mutant AKAP9 proteins markedly diminished the interaction with KCNQ1 subunits, resulting in a reduction of PKA-dependent phosphorylation and in a reduced cAMP-dependent increase of I_{Ks} amplitude.[112]

The *KCNE2* gene on chromosome 21q22 encodes a MinK (LQT-5)-related peptide-1 (MiRP1), a small integral membrane subunit known to assemble experimentally with a plethora of other ion channel subunits (eg, I_{Kr} /KCNH2/LQT-2, I_{Ks}/KCNQ1/LQT-1, I_f/HCN, I_{to} /Kv4.2 and Kv4.3, I_{Kir}/Kv2.1). Gene variation in *KCNE2* has been proposed to be linked to congenital (LQT-6) and to drug-induced forms of LQTS, respectively.[114,115] In this context, variation in the MiRP1 has been shown to alter I_{Kr} channel activity in experimental conditions[114–117]; however, predominant detection of MiRP1 in Purkinje cells rather than in ventricular cardiomyocytes raised questions about the potential role of MiRP1 in myocardial repolarization and, in consequence, in LQTS and in drug-induced LQTS.[118–120]

Rare Sodium Channel-Related Subforms

These subforms include mutations in the gene encoding α1-syntrophin (*STNA1*, chromosome 20q11.21; LQT-12), caveolin 3 (*CAV3*, chromosome 3p25.3; LQT-9), and a β-subunit of the cardiac sodium channel (*SCN4β*; chromosome 11q23.3; LQT-10). Similarly to the main sodium channel-related subform (LQT-3, caused by mutations in the α-subunit), missense mutations in these 3 genes are capable of increasing the late I_{Na} current[121–125] (gain of function) as seen for *SCN5A* (LQT-3) gene mutations. So far, only a single reports exists and does not allow particular phenotypic features of these subforms to be defined. However, the phenotype of a family with LQT-10 resembles that of LQT-3, including QT prolongation and late appearance of T-waves, intermittent (functional) 2:1 atrioventricular block, and T-wave alternans. The β-subunit of the sodium channel has an important role in regulating channel kinetics, signal transduction, and expression of the α-subunit of the sodium channel. In contrast, mutations in the *CAV3* gene (MIM 601253) are typically seen in heritable muscle disorders such as limb-girdle muscular dystrophy (type IC), distal myopathy, rippling muscle disease and increased serum creatine kinase levels.[126]

Other Rare LQTS Subforms

The LQT-4 gene has been mapped to human chromosome 4q25-q27 and is linked to mutations in the *ANK2* (*ANKB*, ankyrin-B) gene. To date, there are only a few reports on *ANK2* mutations[88,127] and, in a targeted analysis, an overall mutation frequency of lower than 5% in otherwise nongenotyped LQTS (ie, non–LQT-13 and non–LQT-56) probands has been reported.[128] Ankyrins, including ankyrin-B, are a protein family that link integral membrane proteins to the underlying spectrin-actin cytoskeleton.[129] In consequence, they play a key role in cell motility, activation, proliferation, and cell-cell contact and in the functional maintenance of specialized membrane domains. Typically, they contain an amino-terminal domain containing multiple ankyrin repeats, a central region with a highly conserved spectrin-binding domain, and a carboxy-terminal regulatory domain. So far, only loss-of-function *ANK2* mutations caused by nonsynonymous amino acid changes have been described.[88,127,128,130] As a clinically recognizable hallmark, *ANK2* mutation carriers showed a distinct spectrum of ECG abnormalities apart from QT interval prolongation; some showed exercise-induced, polymorphic ventricular arrhythmias, sinus bradycardia and prominent U-waves, and atrioventricular conduction block but also syncope, atrial and ventricular fibrillation, and sudden cardiac death. Functionally, ANKB mutants were shown to reduce the cellular localization and protein levels of NCX (an Na/Ca exchanger protein), sodium-potassium ATPase, and IP_3 receptor, and thereby to disrupt cellular functional organization and, in addition, intracellular Ca^{2+} signaling.[130] In a targeted mutation analysis of the last 10 exons (36–46, except 38) covering the C-terminal part of the protein, putative *ANK2* variants have been described in 6 unrelated patients with LQTS, including 3 with other, typical LQTS mutations. In addition, a widespread occurrence of nonsynonymous, polymorphic variants is known from analysis of healthy controls.[128]

LQTS (WITH EXTRACARDIAC MANIFESTATIONS)
Jervell and Lange-Nielsen Syndrome

Homozygous mutations in the 2 LQTS genes encoding subunits for the I_{Ks} potassium channel (LQT-1: *KCNQ1*, and LQT-5: *KCNE1*, respectively), are responsible for Jervell and Lange-Nielsen syndrome (JLNS) (MIM 220400 and 607542).[131] It is an autosomal recessive form of LQTS and associated with congenital inner ear deafness. The 2 subforms, *JLN-1* (KCNQ1 related)[132,133] and JLN-2 (KCNE1 related)[134,135] have a relative ratio of 9:1. Because of the presence of 2 diallelic mutations, JLNS is characterized by a severe QTc prolongation (usually >550 milliseconds) and a high rate of sudden cardiac death.[136,137] The JLN-1 subtype has more a more severe phenotypic expression than subtype JLN-2. In addition to the ECG alteration, the deafness that is caused by an impaired control of endolymph secretions in the inner ear shows a variable phenotypic pattern, even in carriers of 2 I_{Ks} channel gene mutations.[138,139] JLNS occurs in 0.0003% of children and in 1% to 7% of patients with LQTS. Most patients have a consanguineous background; in approximately 10%, compound heterozygosity in 1 of the 2 I_{KS} channel genes is found. Parents of JLNS probands usually show no, or slight, signs of LQTS. However, there is often a family history of sudden death in the young relations.

Andersen-Tawil Syndrome (LQT-7)

Andersen-Tawil syndrome (ATS; MIM 170390) is a rare, autosomal dominant channelopathy[140] with an estimated prevalence of 1:1,000,000. ATS is characterized by episodic attacks of periodic paralysis without myotonia (K+ sensitive; often after exercise or carbohydrate meals, lasting for several hours), QT interval prolongation (not excessive), and evident U-waves, polymorphic ventricular arrhythmias (often unrelated to exercise), and distinctive dysmorphic skeletal features including mandibular hypoplasia (micrognathia), hypertelorism (wide interpupillary distance), low-set ears, broad-based nose, clinodactyly, syndactyly (toes), and small hands and feet.[141–143] Microcephaly and a high-arched palate have also been described. Some patients may have isolated cardiac involvement,[144] and others also show unilateral dysplastic kidney and valvular malformations. The variability in clinical expression can lead to a diagnostic delay because some individuals may have the typical triad phenotype.

Most patients with ATS have a single, heterozygous mutation in the potassium channel gene *KCNJ2* on chromosome 17q24.3 (LQT-7),[145,146] which encodes a major subunit of the inward rectifier K+ channel (I_{K1} current; Kir2.1) and provides repolarization forces during the terminal phase of the cardiac action potential and controls the diastolic membrane potential. I_{K1} channels are formed by coassembly of various Kir2.x proteins (Kir2.1, Kir2.2, and Kir2.3) with Kir2.1 seeming to be the most abundant subtype in ventricular tissue. Until now, about 40 different mutations have been identified in ATS; however, only half of typical patients with ATS may have a *KCNJ2* mutation. In a large kindred with the *KCNJ2* mutation R67W, a sex-specific manifestation (women predominantly cardiac, men predominantly a muscular phenotype) was reported.[141]

In the *KCNJ2* gene, mutant amino acid residues are widely distributed throughout the predicted channel protein; more than 80% of mutations are nonsynonymous amino acid exchanges. In line with the prolonged myocardial repolarization, heterologous expression experiments showed a reduction of I_{K1} currents when ATS mutant K+ channels (LQT-7) were analyzed.[145] These effects were caused by a dominant negative effect of mutant on wild-type protein, impaired PIP_2 binding properties, or by a trafficking defect and, thereby, a quantitative loss of channel function.[145,147–149] A ex vivo study on isolated, muscular ATS tissue showed no gross difference in morphology and differentiation compared with the wild type. Similar to in vitro data from heterologous models, absence of an inwardly rectifying barium-sensitive (I_{K1}-like) current was noted in myotubes with mutant I_{K1} channels and the resting membrane potential was shifted toward depolarizing potentials, thus explaining similar pathophysiologic consequences ex vivo.[150]

Gain-of-function mutations in *KCNJ2* have recently been associated with other inherited arrhythmia phenotypes, such as short QT syndrome (SQT-3)[151,152] or familial atrial fibrillation.[153]

Timothy Syndrome (LQT-8)

Timothy syndrome (TS; MIM 601005) is another rare variant of congenital LQTS that is characterized by QT interval prolongation and additional multiorgan involvement. So far, only a few reports[154–157] exist that describe a variable, extracardiac phenotypic pattern with syndactyly (fingers, toes; 100%); baldness at birth (100%) and dysmorphic facial features ($\sim$50%) including a round face, flat nasal bridge, small upper jaw, low-set ears, or small or misplaced teeth (100%). Many of the surviving children showed developmental delays consistent with language, motor, and generalized cognitive impairment, and autistic features (60%). In the largest series reported so far,[158] the cardiac phenotype included congenital heart malformations (eg, patent ductus arteriosus [59%], patent foramen ovale, ventricular septal defects, and tetralogy of Fallot), transient 2:1 atrioventricular block, and a high rate of sudden death (59%) in the first decade of life.

Because TS is mainly a sporadic disorder, a candidate gene approach was used and unraveled mutations in the α-subunit of the voltage-gated, L-type calcium channel (LTCC; CaV1.2) gene *CACNA1c* (LQT-8) on the human chromosome 12p13.3 is so far the only known cause. The complexity of the syndrome is reflected by the ubiquitous expression of the LTCC in various tissues and the presence of several isoforms; in isoforms containing exon 8A (eg, isoform 18), Splawski and colleagues[158] identified a recurrent, heterozygous missense mutation (G406R) as the definite cause in unrelated patients with TS. The mutant allele was transmitted from the unaffected mother (it is not a germline, but a somatic mosaic carrier, eg, in oral mucosa) to 2 affected children.[158] The degree of mosaicism can vary between tissues; in another report, the G406R mutation was again reported to be associated with a variable, less severe phenotype (syndactyly; normal cognition, QTc 480 milliseconds without cardiac symptoms).[159] Apart from G406R, only 2 other missense mutations (G402S in exon 8, and A1473G, respectively) were seen in patients with TS.[156,160] *CACNA1c* gene mutations in patients with nonsyndromic, congenital LQTS have not yet been noted, but 2 loss-of-function mutations (A39V, G490R) were recently found in patients with ventricular fibrillation, early repolarization disturbances, and a Brugada ECG pattern.[161]

Early functional studies in zebra fish revealed that, in the embryonic lethal phenotype island beat (isl), a loss of L-type calcium currents influenced heart formation and function.[162] The TS mutation G406R mutation was recently one of the first to be investigated, having been obtained after the reprogramming of a patient's fibroblasts into induced pluripotent stem cells (iPS) and the transdifferentiation into human cardiomyocytelike cells.[163] These cells revealed irregular contractions, excess calcium influx, prolonged action potentials and delayed afterdepolarizations, and irregular, spontaneously occurring electrical activity.

Functional analysis in heterologous expression systems revealed that CaV1.2 G406R and G402S both act as gain-of-function mutations and produced maintained and inward depolarizing calcium currents by causing nearly complete loss of voltage-dependent channel inactivation.[158,160] The mutant LTCCs are likely to have a more stabilized open-channel state by disrupting the domain-specific coupling of activation and inactivation[164] that was proposed through altered interaction with an LTCC anchoring protein (AKAP150).[165] These results further prepare the way for antiadrenergic and calcium channel blocking agents in patients with TS.[163,166,167]

UNCLASSIFIED GENETIC SUBFORMS AFTER ROUTINE SEQUENCING

Even after thorough analysis of known LQTS genes, a causal gene mutation may not be detected in a patient with a definite diagnosis. Currently, comprehensive genetic testing may still result in 20% to 25% of patients with LQTS receiving an uninformative result.[168] Overall, unknown genetic heterogeneity exists in LQTS and some patients, in particular those with exercise-induced QT prolongation, might resemble phenocopies of related arrhythmic syndromes[169] or cardiomyopathies. Additional factors may also account for nongenotyping in LQTS genes.

First, other than germline mutations may account for congenital LQTS, such as somatic LQTS gene mutations. Current information is indicative, but still incomplete.[170] Second, mutations in regions relevant for (eg, ion channel) gene regulation or mRNA splicing (evident or cryptic sites) may lead to altered protein levels or composition. Such regions have not been investigated and reported systematically.[171,172] Specific nucleic acid changes in the LQT-1 gene *KCNQ1* (c. 1032 G>A or c. 1032 G>C) initially were not predicted to alter the last amino acid of exon 6 (p. A341A), but were eventually shown to result in aberrant mRNA splicing and exon skipping.[173] Third, larger rearrangements at LQTS gene loci might be undetectable by using conventional polymerase chain reaction amplification techniques. A few results addressing copy-number variation (CNV) of LQTS genes by using alternative techniques (eg, MLPA, high-density single-nucleotide polymorphism arrays) are available and indicate that CNVs might account for 3% to 5% of patients with LQTS without previously having a demonstrated mutation after direct sequencing of major LQTS genes.[174–178]

POSTMORTEM INVESTIGATIONS OF LQTS GENES

Between 5% and 20% of victims of sudden cardiac death (SCD) have a structurally normal heart, and so the cause of death remains unexplained in adults (for review, see Refs.[179,180]). Inherited forms of a primary electrical heart disease such as LQTS are a possible cause for this type of SCD, in particular in the absence of autopsy findings in the heart and in sudden infant death syndrome (SIDS) cases.[181] After initial reports,[182–185] smaller series showed an LQTS gene mutation detection rate in the range of 5% to 15% of cases previously assigned as genuine SIDS[186–188] and as sudden unexpected death in

epilepsy (SUDEP).[189,190] To date, gene mutations in the major LQTS genes, in particular *SCN5A* (LQT-3) and *KCNH2* (LQT-2), but less common in *GPD1L*, *CAV3* (LQT-9), sodium channel β-subunit genes, and *Ryr2* (CPVT-1),[191] have been described in SIDS.

In other patients with sudden unexplained death (SUD) before 50 years of age, cardiologic and genetic examination in surviving relatives was recently shown to reveal the cause of death in 33% of families with SUD (n = 140), including 45 (96%) cases of inherited cardiac diseases. Among them, a primary electrical disease was present in all (100%) cases with SUD before 14 years of age and in nearly 60% of SUD cases between 30 and 49 years of age[192]; LQTS syndrome (19%) was the most prevalent diagnosis. In addition, sudden death during swimming might be related to congenital LQTS (in particular LQT-1)[40,193,194] or CPVT-1; in one-third of victims, a primary electrical heart disease can be identified after molecular autopsy.[44] In another prospective study of autopsy, DNA from 33 SUD victims (median age 25 years), most died during sleep or at rest; in 15% of cases a retrospectively identified LQTS gene mutation and family investigations indicated the probable cause of death.[195]

In the study by Behr and colleagues,[196] 57 SUD victims were investigated with molecular autopsy and by family investigations; a history of additional unexplained premature sudden death was positive in 30% and in 53%, comparable with other studies,[197] an inheritable heart disease ([LQTS, 43%) was diagnosed. For these reasons, a molecular autopsy including genetic testing of cardiac ion channel genes and a detailed familial investigation of SUD or SCD victims should be performed, as recommended recently.[180,198]

REFERENCES

1. Schwartz PJ, Stramba-Badiale M. Repolarization abnormalities in the newborn. J Cardiovasc Pharmacol 2010;55(6):539–43.
2. Schwartz PJ, Stramba-Badiale M, Crotti L, et al. Prevalence of the congenital long-QT syndrome. Circulation 2009;120(18):1761–7.
3. Hayashi K, Fujino N, Uchiyama K, et al. Long QT syndrome and associated gene mutation carriers in Japanese children: results from ECG screening examination. Clin Sci (Lond) 2009;117(12):415–24.
4. Kobza R, Roos M, Niggli B, et al. Prevalence of long and short QT in a young population of 41,767 predominantly male Swiss conscripts. Heart Rhythm 2009;6(5):652–7.
5. Brink PA, Crotti L, Corfield V, et al. Phenotypic variability and unusual clinical severity of congenital

long-QT syndrome in a founder population. Circulation 2005;112(17):2602–10.

6. Marjamaa A, Salomaa V, Newton-Cheh C, et al. High prevalence of four long QT syndrome founder mutations in the Finnish population. Ann Med 2009; 41(3):234–40.

7. Piippo K, Swan H, Pasternack M, et al. A founder mutation of the potassium channel KCNQ1 in long QT syndrome - implications for estimation of disease prevalence and molecular diagnostics. J Am Coll Cardiol 2001;37(2):562–8.

8. Wang Q, Curran ME, Splawski I, et al. Positional cloning of a novel potassium channel gene: KVLQT1 mutations cause cardiac arrhythmias. Nat Genet 1996;12(1):17–23.

9. Winbo A, Diamant UB, Rydberg A, et al. Origin of the Swedish long QT syndrome Y111C/KCNQ1 founder mutation. Heart Rhythm 2011; 8(4):541–7.

10. Itoh H, Shimizu W, Hayashi K, et al. Long QT syndrome with compound mutations is associated with a more severe phenotype: a Japanese multicenter study. Heart Rhythm 2010;7(10):1411–8.

11. Yamaguchi M, Shimizu M, Ino H, et al. Compound heterozygosity for mutations Asp611–>Tyr in KCNQ1 and Asp609–>Gly in KCNH2 associated with severe long QT syndrome. Clin Sci (Lond) 2005;108(2):143–50.

12. Splawski I, Westenskow P, Timothy K, et al. Compound mutations - a common cause of severe Long QT syndrome. Circulation 2003;108(17):182.

13. Larsen LA, Fosdal I, Andersen PS, et al. Recessive Romano-Ward syndrome associated with compound heterozygosity for two mutations in the KVLQT1 gene. Eur J Hum Genet 1999;7(6): 724–8.

14. Ackerman MJ, Splawski I, Makielski JC, et al. Spectrum and prevalence of cardiac sodium channel variants among black, white, Asian, and Hispanic individuals: implications for arrhythmogenic susceptibility and Brugada/long QT syndrome genetic testing. Heart Rhythm 2004;1(5): 600–7.

15. Ackerman MJ, Tester DJ, Jones GS, et al. Ethnic differences in cardiac potassium channel variants: implications for genetic susceptibility to sudden cardiac death and genetic testing for congenital long QT syndrome. Mayo Clin Proc 2003;78(12): 1479–87.

16. Wang Q, Shen J, Splawski I, et al. SCN5A mutations associated with an inherited cardiac arrhythmia, long QT syndrome. Cell 1995;80(5): 805–11.

17. Makita N, Behr E, Shimizu W, et al. The E1784K mutation in SCN5A is associated with mixed clinical phenotype of type 3 long QT syndrome. J Clin Invest 2008;118(6):2219–29.

18. Takehara N, Makita N, Kawabe J, et al. A cardiac sodium channel mutation identified in Brugada syndrome associated with atrial standstill. J Intern Med 2004;255(1):137–42.

19. Huang H, Zhao J, Barrane FZ, et al. Nav1.5/R1193Q polymorphism is associated with both long QT and Brugada syndromes. Can J Cardiol 2006;22(4):309–13.

20. Hwang HW, Chen JJ, Lin YJ, et al. R1193Q of SCN5A, a Brugada and long QT mutation, is a common polymorphism in Han Chinese. J Med Genet 2005;42(2):e7.

21. Makielski JC, Ye B, Valdivia CR, et al. A ubiquitous splice variant and a common polymorphism affect heterologous expression of recombinant human SCN5A heart sodium channels. Circ Res 2003; 93(9):821–8.

22. Niu DM, Hwang B, Hwang HW, et al. A common SCN5A polymorphism attenuates a severe cardiac phenotype caused by a nonsense SCN5A mutation in a Chinese family with an inherited cardiac conduction defect. J Med Genet 2006;43(10): 817–21.

23. Olszak-Waskiewicz M, Kubik L, Dziuk M, et al. The association between SCN5A, KCNQ1 and KCNE1 gene polymorphisms and complex ventricular arrhythmias in survivors of myocardial infarction. Kardiol Pol 2008;66(8):845–53.

24. Poelzing S, Forleo C, Samodell M, et al. SCN5A polymorphism restores trafficking of a Brugada syndrome mutation on a separate gene. Circulation 2006;114(5):368–76.

25. Tan BH, Valdivia CR, Rok BA, et al. Common human SCN5A polymorphisms have altered electrophysiology when expressed in Q1077 splice variants. Heart Rhythm 2005;2(7): 741–7.

26. Viswanathan PC, Benson DW, Balser JR. A common SCN5A polymorphism modulates the biophysical effects of an SCN5A mutation. J Clin Invest 2003;111(3):341–6.

27. Ye B, Ackerman MJ, Makielski JC. SCN5A can serve as its own modifier - a trafficking defective SCN5A arrhythmia mutation, M1766L, is corrected by the common polymorphism H558R. Circulation 2002;106(19):225.

28. Splawski I, Timothy KW, Tateyama M, et al. Variant of SCN5A sodium channel implicated in risk of cardiac arrhythmia. Science 2002;297(5585): 1333–6.

29. Kapa S, Tester DJ, Salisbury BA, et al. Genetic testing for long-QT syndrome: distinguishing pathogenic mutations from benign variants. Circulation 2009;120(18):1752–60.

30. Schwartz PJ, Moss AJ, Vincent GM, et al. Diagnostic criteria for the long QT syndrome. An update. Circulation 1993;88(2):782–4.

31. Rautaharju PM, Surawicz B, Gettes LS, et al. AHA/ ACCF/HRS recommendations for the standardization and interpretation of the electrocardiogram: part IV: the ST segment, T and U waves, and the QT interval: a scientific statement from the American Heart Association Electrocardiography and Arrhythmias Committee, Council on Clinical Cardiology; the American College of Cardiology Foundation; and the Heart Rhythm Society. Endorsed by the International Society for Computerized Electrocardiology. J Am Coll Cardiol 2009;53(11): 982–91.

32. Chiang AY, Bass AS, Cooper MM, et al. ILSI-HESI cardiovascular safety subcommittee dataset: an analysis of the statistical properties of QT interval and rate-corrected QT interval (QTc). J Pharmacol Toxicol Methods 2007;56(2):95–102.

33. Ackerman MJ, Priori SG, Willems S, et al. HRS/ EHRA expert consensus statement on the state of genetic testing for the channelopathies and cardiomyopathies: this document was developed as a partnership between the Heart Rhythm Society (HRS) and the European Heart Rhythm Association (EHRA). Heart Rhythm 2011;8(8):1308–39.

34. Viskin S, Sands A, Seltzer D, et al. Too many physicians cannot recognize a long QT when they see one. Circulation 2003;108(17):426.

35. Wilde AA, Brugada R. Phenotypical manifestations of mutations in the genes encoding subunits of the cardiac sodium channel. Circ Res 2011;108(7): 884–97.

36. Goldenberg I, Thottathil P, Lopes CM, et al. Trigger-specific ion-channel mechanisms, risk factors, and response to therapy in type 1 long QT syndrome. Heart Rhythm 2012;9(1):49–56.

37. Darbar D. Triggers for cardiac events in patients with type 2 long QT syndrome. Heart Rhythm 2010;7(12):1806–7.

38. Kim JA, Lopes CM, Moss AJ, et al. Trigger-specific risk factors and response to therapy in long QT syndrome type 2. Heart Rhythm 2010;7(12): 1797–805.

39. Sakaguchi T, Shimizu W, Itoh H, et al. Age- and genotype-specific triggers for life-threatening arrhythmia in the genotyped long QT syndrome. J Cardiovasc Electrophysiol 2008;19(8):794–9.

40. Schwartz PJ, Priori SG, Spazzolini C, et al. Genotype-phenotype correlation in the long-QT syndrome: gene-specific triggers for life-threatening arrhythmias. Circulation 2001;103(1):89–95.

41. Jons C, Uchi J, Moss AJ, et al. Use of mutant-specific ion channel characteristics for risk stratification of long QT syndrome patients. Sci Transl Med 2011;3(76):76ra28.

42. Barsheshet A, Peterson DR, Moss AJ, et al. Genotype-specific QT correction for heart rate and the risk of life threatening cardiac events in adolescents with the congenital long-QT syndrome. Heart Rhythm 2011;8(8):1207–13.

43. Bai R, Napolitano C, Bloise R, et al. Yield of genetic screening in inherited cardiac channelopathies: how to prioritize access to genetic testing. Circ Arrhythm Electrophysiol 2009;2(1):6–15.

44. Kapplinger JD, Tester DJ, Salisbury BA, et al. Spectrum and prevalence of mutations from the first 2,500 consecutive unrelated patients referred for the FAMILION long QT syndrome genetic test. Heart Rhythm 2009;6(9):1297–303.

45. Napolitano C, Priori SG, Schwartz PJ, et al. Genetic testing in the long QT syndrome: development and validation of an efficient approach to genotyping in clinical practice. JAMA 2005;294(23):2975–80.

46. Keating M, Atkinson D, Dunn C, et al. Linkage of a cardiac arrhythmia, the long QT syndrome, and the Harvey ras-1 gene [see comments]. Science 1991;252(5006):704–6.

47. Wedekind H, Burde D, Zumhagen S, et al. QT interval prolongation and risk for cardiac events in genotyped LQTS-index children. Eur J Pediatr 2009;168(9):1107–15.

48. Tan HL, Bardai A, Shimizu W, et al. Genotype-specific onset of arrhythmias in congenital long-QT syndrome: possible therapy implications. Circulation 2006;114(20):2096–103.

49. Crotti L, Spazzolini C, Schwartz PJ, et al. The common long-QT syndrome mutation KCNQ1/ A341V causes unusually severe clinical manifestations in patients with different ethnic backgrounds: toward a mutation-specific risk stratification. Circulation 2007;116(21):2366–75.

50. Mikuni I, Torres CG, Bienengraeber MW, et al. Partial restoration of the long QT syndrome associated KCNQ1 A341V mutant by the KCNE1 beta-subunit. Biochim Biophys Acta 2011;1810(12): 1285–93.

51. Li H, Chen Q, Moss AJ, et al. New mutations in the KVLQT1 potassium channel that cause long-QT syndrome. Circulation 1998;97(13):1264–9.

52. Bartos DC, Duchatelet S, Burgess DE, et al. R231C mutation in KCNQ1 causes long QT syndrome type 1 and familial atrial fibrillation. Heart Rhythm 2011; 8(1):48–55.

53. Lundby A, Ravn LS, Svendsen JH, et al. KCNQ1 mutation Q147R is associated with atrial fibrillation and prolonged QT interval. Heart Rhythm 2007; 4(12):1532–41.

54. Chen S, Zhang L, Bryant RM, et al. KCNQ1 mutations in patients with a family history of lethal cardiac arrhythmias and sudden death. Clin Genet 2003;63(4):273–82.

55. Bellocq C, van Ginneken ACG, Bezzina CR, et al. Mutation in the KCNQ1 gene leading to the short QT-interval syndrome. Circulation 2004;109(20): 2394–7.

56. Imboden M, Swan H, Denjoy I, et al. Female predominance and transmission distortion in the long-QT syndrome. N Engl J Med 2006;355(26): 2744–51.

57. Curran ME, Splawski I, Timothy KW, et al. A molecular basis for cardiac arrhythmia: HERG mutations cause long QT syndrome. Cell 1995; 80(5):795–803.

58. Sanguinetti MC, Jiang C, Curran ME, et al. A mechanistic link between an inherited and an acquired cardiac arrhythmia: HERG encodes the IKr potassium channel. Cell 1995;81(2): 299–307.

59. Biliczki P, Girmatsion Z, Brandes RP, et al. Trafficking-deficient long QT syndrome mutation KCNQ1-T587M confers severe clinical phenotype by impairment of KCNH2 membrane localization: evidence for clinically significant IKr-IKs alpha-subunit interaction. Heart Rhythm 2009;6(12): 1792–801.

60. Ficker E, Thomas D, Viswanathan PC, et al. Novel characteristics of a misprocessed mutant HERG channel linked to hereditary long QT syndrome. Am J Physiol Heart Circ Physiol 2000;279(4): H1748–56.

61. Mihic A, Chauhan VS, Gao X, et al. Trafficking defect and proteasomal degradation contribute to the phenotype of a novel KCNH2 long QT syndrome mutation. PLoS One 2011;6(3):e18273.

62. Anderson CL, Delisle BP, Anson BD, et al. Most LQT2 mutations reduce Kv11.1 (hERG) current by a class 2 (trafficking-deficient) mechanism. Circulation 2006;113(3):365–73.

63. Bhuiyan ZA, Momenah TS, Gong Q, et al. Recurrent intrauterine fetal loss due to near absence of HERG: clinical and functional characterization of a homozygous nonsense HERG Q1070X mutation. Heart Rhythm 2008;5(4):553–61.

64. Hoorntje T, Alders M, van Tintelen P, et al. Homozygous premature truncation of the HERG protein: the human HERG knockout. Circulation 1999;100(12): 1264–7.

65. Johnson WH Jr, Yang P, Yang T, et al. Clinical, genetic, and biophysical characterization of a homozygous HERG mutation causing severe neonatal long QT syndrome. Pediatr Res 2003; 53(5):744–8.

66. Teng GQ, Zhao X, Lees-Miller JP, et al. Homozygous missense N629D hERG (KCNH2) potassium channel mutation causes developmental defects in the right ventricle and its outflow tract and embryonic lethality. Circ Res 2008;103(12): 1483–91.

67. Hong K, Bjerregaard P, Gussak I, et al. Short QT syndrome and atrial fibrillation caused by mutation in KCNH2. J Cardiovasc Electrophysiol 2005;16(4): 394–6.

68. Itoh H, Sakaguchi T, Ashihara T, et al. A novel KCNH2 mutation as a modifier for short QT interval. Int J Cardiol 2009;137(1):83–5.

69. Brugada R, Hong K, Dumaine R, et al. Sudden death associated with short-QT syndrome linked to mutations in HERG. Circulation 2004;109(1): 30–5.

70. Bennett PB, Yazawa K, Makita N, et al. Molecular mechanism for an inherited cardiac arrhythmia. Nature 1995;376(6542):683–5.

71. Zimmer T, Surber R. SCN5A channelopathies–an update on mutations and mechanisms. Prog Biophys Mol Biol 2008;98(2–3):120–36.

72. Clancy CE, Tateyama M, Liu H, et al. Non-equilibrium gating in cardiac Na+ channels: an original mechanism of arrhythmia. Circulation 2003;107(17): 2233–7.

73. Makiyama T, Akao M, Shizuta S, et al. A novel SCN5A gain-of-function mutation M1875T associated with familial atrial fibrillation. J Am Coll Cardiol 2008;52(16):1326–34.

74. Benito B, Brugada R, Perich RM, et al. A mutation in the sodium channel is responsible for the association of long QT syndrome and familial atrial fibrillation. Heart Rhythm 2008;5(10):1434–40.

75. Surber R, Hensellek S, Prochnau D, et al. Combination of cardiac conduction disease and long QT syndrome caused by mutation T1620K in the cardiac sodium channel. Cardiovasc Res 2008; 77(4):740–8.

76. Clancy CE, Rudy Y. Na(+) channel mutation that causes both Brugada and long-QT syndrome phenotypes: a simulation study of mechanism. Circulation 2002;105(10):1208–13.

77. Veldkamp MW, Viswanathan PC, Bezzina C, et al. Two distinct congenital arrhythmias evoked by a multidysfunctional Na(+) channel. Circ Res 2000;86(9):E91–7.

78. Ruan Y, Liu N, Bloise R, et al. Gating properties of SCN5A mutations and the response to mexiletine in long-QT syndrome type 3 patients. Circulation 2007;116(10):1137–44.

79. Shimizu W, Antzelevitch C. Sodium channel block with mexiletine is effective in reducing dispersion of repolarization and preventing torsade des pointes in LQT2 and LQT3 models of the long-QT syndrome. Circulation 1997;96(6):2038–47.

80. Windle JR, Geletka RC, Moss AJ, et al. Normalization of ventricular repolarization with flecainide in long QT syndrome patients with SCN5A: DeltaKPQ mutation. Ann Noninvasive Electrocardiol 2001; 6(2):153–8.

81. Ruan Y, Denegri M, Liu N, et al. Trafficking defects and gating abnormalities of a novel SCN5A mutation question gene-specific therapy in long QT syndrome type 3. Circ Res 2010; 106(8):1374–83.

82. Cheng J, Morales A, Siegfried JD, et al. SCN5A rare variants in familial dilated cardiomyopathy decrease peak sodium current depending on the common polymorphism H558R and common splice variant Q1077del. Clin Transl Sci 2010;3(6): 287–94.

83. Shinlapawittayatorn K, Du XX, Liu H, et al. A common SCN5A polymorphism modulates the biophysical defects of SCN5A mutations. Heart Rhythm 2011;8(3):455–62.

84. Hu D, Viskin S, Oliva A, et al. Novel mutation in the SCN5A gene associated with arrhythmic storm development during acute myocardial infarction. Heart Rhythm 2007;4(8):1072–80.

85. Stecker EC, Sono M, Wallace E, et al. Allelic variants of SCN5A and risk of sudden cardiac arrest in patients with coronary artery disease. Heart Rhythm 2006;3(6):697–700.

86. Tan BH, Valdivia CR, Song C, et al. Partial expression defect for the SCN5A missense mutation G1406R depends on splice variant background Q1077 and rescue by mexiletine. Am J Physiol Heart Circ Physiol 2006;291(4):H1822–8.

87. Schott JJ, Charpentier F, Peltier S, et al. Mapping of a gene for long QT syndrome to chromosome 4q25-27. Am J Hum Genet 1995;57(5):1114–22.

88. Mohler PJ, Schott JJ, Gramolini AO, et al. Ankyrin-B mutation causes type 4 long-QT cardiac arrhythmia and sudden cardiac death. Nature 2003; 421(6923):634–9.

89. Yang Y, Yang Y, Liang B, et al. Identification of a Kir3.4 mutation in congenital long QT syndrome. Am J Hum Genet 2010;86(6):872–80.

90. Sanguinetti MC, Curran ME, Zou A, et al. Coassembly of K(V)LQT1 and minK (IsK) proteins to form cardiac I(Ks) potassium channel. Nature 1996; 384(6604):80–3.

91. Barhanin J, Lesage F, Guillemare E, et al. K(V)LQT1 and IsK (minK) proteins associate to form the I(Ks) cardiac potassium current [see comments]. Nature 1996;384(6604):78–80.

92. Splawski I, Tristani-Firouzi M, Lehmann MH, et al. Mutations in the hminK gene cause long QT syndrome and suppress IKs function. Nat Genet 1997;17(3):338–40.

93. Ohno S, Zankov DP, Yoshida H, et al. N- and C-terminal KCNE1 mutations cause distinct phenotypes of long QT syndrome. Heart Rhythm 2007; 4(3):332–40.

94. Wu DM, Lai LP, Zhang M, et al. Characterization of an LQT5-related mutation in KCNE1, Y81C: implications for a role of KCNE1 cytoplasmic domain in IKs channel function. Heart Rhythm 2006;3(9): 1031–40.

95. Ma L, Lin C, Teng S, et al. Characterization of a novel long QT syndrome mutation G52R-KCNE1 in a Chinese family. Cardiovasc Res 2003;59(3):612–9.

96. Schulze-Bahr E, Schwarz M, Hoffmann S, et al. A novel long-QT 5 gene mutation in the C-terminus (V109I) is associated with a mild phenotype. J Mol Med 2001;79(9):504–9.

97. Duggal P, Vesely MR, Wattanasirichaigoon D, et al. Mutation of the gene for IsK associated with both Jervell and Lange-Nielsen and Romano-Ward forms of Long-QT syndrome. Circulation 1998; 97(2):142–6.

98. Bianchi L, Shen Z, Dennis AT, et al. Cellular dysfunction of LQT5-minK mutants: abnormalities of IKs, IKr and trafficking in long QT syndrome. Hum Mol Genet 1999;8(8):1499–507.

99. Marx SO, Kurokawa J, Reiken S, et al. Requirement of a macromolecular signaling complex for beta adrenergic receptor modulation of the KCNQ1-KCNE1 potassium channel. Science 2002; 295(5554):496–9.

100. Harmer SC, Wilson AJ, Aldridge R, et al. Mechanisms of disease pathogenesis in long QT syndrome type 5. Am J Physiol Cell Physiol 2010; 298(2):C263–73.

101. Zheng R, Thompson K, Obeng-Gyimah E, et al. Analysis of the interactions between the C-terminal cytoplasmic domains of KCNQ1 and KCNE1 channel subunits. Biochem J 2010;428(1):75–84.

102. Chen J, Zheng R, Melman YF, et al. Functional interactions between KCNE1 C-terminus and the KCNQ1 channel. PLoS One 2009;4(4): e5143.

103. Xu X, Jiang M, Hsu KL, et al. KCNQ1 and KCNE1 in the IKs channel complex make state-dependent contacts in their extracellular domains. J Gen Physiol 2008;131(6):589–603.

104. Seebohm G, Strutz-Seebohm N, Ureche ON, et al. Long QT syndrome-associated mutations in KCNQ1 and KCNE1 subunits disrupt normal endosomal recycling of IKs channels. Circ Res 2008;103(12): 1451–7.

105. Seebohm G, Strutz-Seebohm N, Birkin R, et al. Regulation of endocytic recycling of KCNQ1/KCNE1 potassium channels. Circ Res 2007; 100(5):686–92.

106. Harmer SC, Tinker A. The role of abnormal trafficking of KCNE1 in long QT syndrome 5. Biochem Soc Trans 2007;35(Pt 5):1074–6.

107. Li Y, Zaydman MA, Wu D, et al. KCNE1 enhances phosphatidylinositol 4,5-bisphosphate (PIP2) sensitivity of IKs to modulate channel activity. Proc Natl Acad Sci U S A 2011;108(22):9095–100.

108. Melman YF, Um SY, Krumerman A, et al. KCNE1 binds to the KCNQ1 pore to regulate potassium channel activity. Neuron 2004;42(6):927–37.

109. Krapivinsky G, Gordon EA, Wickman K, et al. The G-protein-gated atrial K+ channel IKACh is a heteromultimer of two inwardly rectifying K(+)-channel proteins. Nature 1995;374(6518):135–41.

110. Calloe K, Ravn LS, Schmitt N, et al. Characteriza- tions of a loss-of-function mutation in the Kir3.4 channel subunit. Biochem Biophys Res Commun 2007;364(4):889–95.

111. Choi M, Scholl UI, Yue P, et al. K+ channel mutations in adrenal aldosterone-producing ade- nomas and hereditary hypertension. Science 2011;331(6018):768–72.

112. Chen L, Marquardt ML, Tester DJ, et al. Mutation of an A-kinase-anchoring protein causes long-QT syndrome. Proc Natl Acad Sci U S A 2007; 104(52):20990–5.

113. Kurokawa J, Motoike HK, Rao J, et al. Regulatory actions of the A-kinase anchoring protein Yotiao on a heart potassium channel downstream of PKA phosphorylation. Proc Natl Acad Sci U S A 2004;101(46):16374–8.

114. Sesti F, Abbott GW, Wei J, et al. A common poly- morphism associated with antibiotic-induced car- diac arrhythmia. Proc Natl Acad Sci U S A 2000; 97(19):10613–8.

115. Abbott GW, Sesti F, Splawski I, et al. MiRP1 forms IKr potassium channels with HERG and is associ- ated with cardiac arrhythmia. Cell 1999;97(2): 175–87.

116. Cui J, Kagan A, Qin D, et al. Analysis of the cyclic nucleotide binding domain of the HERG potassium channel and interactions with KCNE2. J Biol Chem 2001;276(20):17244–51.

117. Isbrandt D, Friederich P, Solth A, et al. Identification and functional characterization of a novel KCNE2 (MiRP1) mutation that alters HERG channel kinetics. J Mol Med 2002;80(8):524–32.

118. Pourrier M, Zicha S, Ehrlich J, et al. Canine ventricular KCNE2 expression resides predomi- nantly in Purkinje fibers. Circ Res 2003;93(3): 189–91.

119. Pond AL, Nerbonne JM. ERG proteins and func- tional cardiac I(Kr) channels in rat, mouse, and human heart. Trends Cardiovasc Med 2001;11(7): 286–94.

120. Friederich P, Solth A, Schillemeit S, et al. Local anaesthetic sensitivities of cloned HERG channels from human heart: comparison with HERG/MiRP1 and HERG/MiRP1(T8A). Br J Anaesth 2004;92(1): 93–101.

121. Ueda K, Valdivia C, Medeiros-Domingo A, et al. Syntrophin mutation associated with long QT syndrome through activation of the nNOS-SCN5A macromolecular complex. Proc Natl Acad Sci U S A 2008;105(27):9355–60.

122. Wu G, Ai T, Kim JJ, et al. α-1-Syntrophin mutation and the long-QT syndrome: a disease of sodium channel disruption. Circ Arrhythm Electrophysiol 2008;1(3):193–201.

123. Cronk LB, Ye B, Kaku T, et al. Novel mechanism for sudden infant death syndrome: persistent late

sodium current secondary to mutations in caveo- lin-3. Heart Rhythm 2007;4(2):161–6.

124. Vatta M, Ackerman MJ, Ye B, et al. Mutant caveolin- 3 induces persistent late sodium current and is associated with long-QT syndrome. Circulation 2006;114(20):2104–12.

125. Medeiros-Domingo A, Kaku T, Tester DJ, et al. SCN4B-encoded sodium channel beta4 subunit in congenital long-QT syndrome. Circulation 2007; 116(2):134–42.

126. Gazzerro E, Bonetto A, Minetti C. Caveolinopathies translational implications of caveolin-3 in skeletal and cardiac muscle disorders. Handb Clin Neurol 2011;101:135–42.

127. Mohler PJ, Splawski I, Napolitano C, et al. A cardiac arrhythmia syndrome caused by loss of ankyrin-B function. Proc Natl Acad Sci U S A 2004;101(24):9137–42.

128. Sherman J, Tester DJ, Ackerman MJ. Targeted mutational analysis of ankyrin-B in 541 consecu- tive, unrelated patients referred for long QT syndrome genetic testing and 200 healthy subjects. Heart Rhythm 2005;2(11):1218–23.

129. Curran J, Mohler PJ. Coordinating electrical activity of the heart: ankyrin polypeptides in human cardiac disease. Expert Opin Ther Targets 2011; 15(7):789–801.

130. Mohler PJ, Le Scouarnec S, Denjoy I, et al. Defining the cellular phenotype of "ankyrin-B syndrome" variants: human ANK2 variants associ- ated with clinical phenotypes display a spectrum of activities in cardiomyocytes. Circulation 2007; 115(4):432–41.

131. Jervell A, Lange-Nielsen F. Congenital deaf- mutism, functional heart disease with prolongation of the Q-T interval and sudden death. Am Heart J 1957;54(1):59–68.

132. Chen Q, Zhang D, Gingell RL, et al. Homozygous deletion in KVLQT1 associated with Jervell and Lange-Nielsen syndrome. Circulation 1999;99(10): 1344–7.

133. Neyroud N, Tesson F, Denjoy I, et al. A novel muta- tion in the potassium channel gene KVLQT1 causes the Jervell and Lange-Nielsen cardioaudi- tory syndrome [see comments]. Nat Genet 1997; 15(2):186–9.

134. Schulze-Bahr E, Wang Q, Wedekind H, et al. KCNE1 mutations cause Jervell and Lange- Nielsen syndrome. Nat Genet 1997;17(3):267–8.

135. Tyson J, Tranebjaerg L, Bellman S, et al. IsK and KvLQT1: mutation in either of the two subunits of the slow component of the delayed rectifier potas- sium channel can cause Jervell and Lange- Nielsen syndrome. Hum Mol Genet 1997;6(12): 2179–85.

136. Schwartz PJ, Spazzolini C, Crotti L, et al. The Jer- vell and Lange-Nielsen syndrome: natural history,

molecular basis, and clinical outcome. Circulation 2006;113(6):783–90.

137. Goldenberg I, Moss AJ, Zareba W, et al. Clinical course and risk stratification of patients affected with the Jervell and Lange-Nielsen syndrome. J Cardiovasc Electrophysiol 2006;17(11): 1161–8.

138. Zhang S, Yin K, Ren X, et al. Identification of a novel KCNQ1 mutation associated with both Jervell and Lange-Nielsen and Romano-Ward forms of long QT syndrome in a Chinese family. BMC Med Genet 2008;9:24.

139. Bhuiyan ZA, Momenah TS, Amin AS, et al. An intronic mutation leading to incomplete skipping of exon-2 in KCNQ1 rescues hearing in Jervell and Lange-Nielsen syndrome. Prog Biophys Mol Biol 2008;98(2–3):319–27.

140. Tawil R, Ptacek LJ, Pavlakis SG, et al. Andersen's syndrome: potassium-sensitive periodic paralysis, ventricular ectopy, and dysmorphic features [see comments]. Ann Neurol 1994;35(3):326–30.

141. Andelfinger G, Tapper AR, Welch RC, et al. KCNJ2 mutation results in Andersen syndrome with sex-specific cardiac and skeletal muscle phenotypes. Am J Hum Genet 2002;71(3):663–8.

142. Davies NP, Imbrici P, Fialho D, et al. Andersen-Tawil syndrome: new potassium channel mutations and possible phenotypic variation. Neurology 2005; 65(7):1083–9.

143. Yoon G, Quitania L, Kramer JH, et al. Andersen-Tawil syndrome: definition of a neurocognitive phenotype. Neurology 2006;66(11):1703–10.

144. Fodstad HM, Swan H, Auberson M, et al. Mutations in the potassium channel gene KCNJ2 constitute a rare cause of long QT syndrome. Am J Hum Genet 2003;73(5):557.

145. Tristani-Firouzi M, Jensen JL, Donaldson MR, et al. Functional and clinical characterization of KCNJ2 mutations associated with LQT7 (Andersen syndrome). J Clin Invest 2002;110(3):381–8.

146. Plaster NM, Tawil R, Tristani-Firouzi M, et al. Mutations in Kir2.1 cause the developmental and episodic electrical phenotypes of Andersen's syndrome. Cell 2001;105(4):511–9.

147. Doi T, Makiyama T, Morimoto T, et al. A novel KCNJ2 nonsense mutation, S369X, impedes trafficking and causes a limited form of Andersen-Tawil syndrome. Circ Cardiovasc Genet 2011; 4(3):253–60.

148. Donaldson MR, Jensen JL, Tristani-Firouzi M, et al. PIP2 binding residues of Kir2.1 are common targets of mutations causing Andersen syndrome. Neurology 2003;60(11):1811–6.

149. Haruna Y, Kobori A, Makiyama T, et al. Genotype-phenotype correlations of KCNJ2 mutations in Japanese patients with Andersen-Tawil syndrome. Hum Mutat 2007;28(2):208.

150. Sacconi S, Simkin D, Arrighi N, et al. Mechanisms underlying Andersen's syndrome pathology in skeletal muscle are revealed in human myotubes. Am J Physiol Cell Physiol 2009;297(4):C876–85.

151. Priori SG, Pandit SV, Rivolta I, et al. A novel form of short QT syndrome (SQT3) is caused by a mutation in the KCNJ2 gene. Circ Res 2005;96(7):800–7.

152. Hattori T, Makiyama T, Akao M, et al. A novel gain-of-function KCNJ2 mutation associated with short QT syndrome impairs inward rectification of Kir2.1 currents. Cardiovasc Res 2011. [Epub ahead of print].

153. Xia M, Jin Q, Bendahhou S, et al. A Kir2.1 gain-of-function mutation underlies familial atrial fibrillation. Biochem Biophys Res Commun 2005;332(4): 1012–9.

154. Reichenbach H, Meister EM, Theile H. The heart-hand syndrome. A new variant of disorders of heart conduction and syndactylia including osseous changes in hands and feet. Kinderarztl Prax 1992;60(2):54–6 [in German].

155. Marks ML, Whisler SL, Clericuzio C, et al. A new form of long QT syndrome associated with syndactyly. J Am Coll Cardiol 1995;25(1):59–64.

156. Gillis J, Burashnikov E, Antzelevitch C, et al. Long QT, syndactyly, joint contractures, stroke and novel CACNA1C mutation: expanding the spectrum of Timothy syndrome. Am J Med Genet A 2011. [Epub ahead of print].

157. Krause U, Gravenhorst V, Kriebel T, et al. A rare association of long QT syndrome and syndactyly: Timothy syndrome (LQT 8). Clin Res Cardiol 2011;100(12):1123–7.

158. Splawski I, Timothy KW, Sharpe LM, et al. Ca(V)1.2 calcium channel dysfunction causes a multisystem disorder including arrhythmia and autism. Cell 2004;119(1):19–31.

159. Etheridge SP, Bowles NE, Arrington CB, et al. Somatic mosaicism contributes to phenotypic variation in Timothy syndrome. Am J Med Genet A 2011;155(10):2578–83.

160. Splawski I, Timothy KW, Decher N, et al. Severe arrhythmia disorder caused by cardiac L-type calcium channel mutations. Proc Natl Acad Sci U S A 2005;102(23):8089–96.

161. Antzelevitch C, Pollevick GD, Cordeiro JM, et al. Loss-of-function mutations in the cardiac calcium channel underlie a new clinical entity characterized by ST-segment elevation, short QT intervals, and sudden cardiac death. Circulation 2007;115(4):442–9.

162. Rottbauer W, Baker K, Wo ZG, et al. Growth and function of the embryonic heart depend upon the cardiac-specific L-type calcium channel alpha1 subunit. Dev Cell 2001;1(2):265–75.

163. Yazawa M, Hsueh B, Jia X, et al. Using induced pluripotent stem cells to investigate cardiac phenotypes in Timothy syndrome. Nature 2011; 471(7337):230–4.

164. Depil K, Beyl S, Stary-Weinzinger A, et al. Timothy mutation disrupts the link between activation and inactivation in Ca(V)1.2 protein. J Biol Chem 2011;286(36):31557–64.

165. Cheng EP, Yuan C, Navedo MF, et al. Restoration of normal L-type Ca2+ channel function during timothy syndrome by ablation of an anchoring protein. Circ Res 2011;109(3):255–61.

166. Jacobs A, Knight BP, McDonald KT, et al. Verapamil decreases ventricular tachyarrhythmias in a patient with Timothy syndrome (LQT8). Heart Rhythm 2006;3(8):967–70.

167. Yarotskyy V, Gao G, Peterson BZ, et al. The Timothy syndrome mutation of cardiac CaV1.2 (L-type) channels: multiple altered gating mechanisms and pharmacological restoration of inactivation. J Physiol 2009;587(Pt 3):551–65.

168. Tester DJ, Ackerman MJ. Genetic testing for potentially lethal, highly treatable inherited cardiomyopathies/channelopathies in clinical practice. Circulation 2011;123(9):1021–37.

169. Medeiros-Domingo A, Bhuiyan ZA, Tester DJ, et al. The RYR2-encoded ryanodine receptor/calcium release channel in patients diagnosed previously with either catecholaminergic polymorphic ventricular tachycardia or genotype negative, exercise-induced long QT syndrome: a comprehensive open reading frame mutational analysis. J Am Coll Cardiol 2009;54(22):2065–74.

170. Miller TE, Estrella E, Myerburg RJ, et al. Recurrent third-trimester fetal loss and maternal mosaicism for long-QT syndrome. Circulation 2004;109(24): 3029–34.

171. Crotti L, Lewandowska MA, Schwartz PJ, et al. A KCNH2 branch point mutation causing aberrant splicing contributes to an explanation of genotype-negative long QT syndrome. Heart Rhythm 2009;6(2):212–8.

172. Zhang L, Vincent GM, Baralle M, et al. An intronic mutation causes long QT syndrome. J Am Coll Cardiol 2004;44(6):1283–91.

173. Murray A, Donger C, Fenske C, et al. Splicing mutations in KCNQ1: a mutation hot spot at codon 344 that produces in frame transcripts. Circulation 1999;100(10):1077–84.

174. Barc J, Briec F, Schmitt S, et al. Screening for copy number variation in genes associated with the long QT syndrome: clinical relevance. J Am Coll Cardiol 2011;57(1):40–7.

175. Grilo LS, Pruvot E, Grobety M, et al. Takotsubo cardiomyopathy and congenital long QT syndrome in a patient with a novel duplication in the Per-Arnt-Sim (PAS) domain of hERG1. Heart Rhythm 2010; 7(2):260–5.

176. Koopmann TT, Alders M, Jongbloed RJ, et al. Long QT syndrome caused by a large duplication in the KCNH2 (HERG) gene undetectable by current polymerase chain reaction-based exon-scanning methodologies. Heart Rhythm 2006;3(1):52–5.

177. Eddy CA, MacCormick JM, Chung SK, et al. Identification of large gene deletions and duplications in KCNQ1 and KCNH2 in patients with long QT syndrome. Heart Rhythm 2008;5(9):1275–81.

178. Tester DJ, Benton AJ, Train L, et al. Prevalence and spectrum of large deletions or duplications in the major long QT syndrome-susceptibility genes and implications for long QT syndrome genetic testing. Am J Cardiol 2010;106(8):1124–8.

179. Oliva A, Brugada R, D'Aloja E, et al. State of the art in forensic investigation of sudden cardiac death. Am J Forensic Med Pathol 2011;32(1):1–16.

180. Basso C, Carturan E, Pilichou K, et al. Sudden cardiac death with normal heart: molecular autopsy. Cardiovasc Pathol 2010;19(6):321–5.

181. Opdal SH, Rognum TO. Gene variants predisposing to SIDS: current knowledge. Forensic Sci Med Pathol 2011;7(1):26–36.

182. Schwartz PJ, Priori SG, Dumaine R, et al. A molecular link between the sudden infant death syndrome and the long-QT syndrome. N Engl J Med 2000;343(4):262–7.

183. Schwartz PJ, Priori SG, Bloise R, et al. Molecular diagnosis in a child with sudden infant death syndrome. Lancet 2001;358(9290):1342–3.

184. Wedekind H, Smits JP, Schulze-Bahr E, et al. De novo mutation in the SCN5A gene associated with early onset of sudden infant death. Circulation 2001;104(10):1158–64.

185. Aurlien D, Leren TP, Tauboll E, et al. New SCN5A mutation in a SUDEP victim with idiopathic epilepsy. Seizure 2009;18(2):158–60.

186. Arnestad M, Crotti L, Rognum TO, et al. Prevalence of long-QT syndrome gene variants in sudden infant death syndrome. Circulation 2007;115(3):361–7.

187. Wedekind H, Bajanowski T, Friederich P, et al. Sudden infant death syndrome and long QT syndrome: an epidemiological and genetic study. Int J Legal Med 2006;120(3):129–37.

188. Ackerman MJ, Siu BL, Sturner WQ, et al. Postmortem molecular analysis of SCN5A defects in sudden infant death syndrome. JAMA 2001; 286(18):2264–9.

189. Tu E, Bagnall RD, Duflou J, et al. Post-mortem review and genetic analysis of sudden unexpected death in epilepsy (SUDEP) cases. Brain Pathol 2011;21(2):201–8.

190. Johnson JN, Hofman N, Haglund CM, et al. Identification of a possible pathogenic link between congenital long QT syndrome and epilepsy. Neurology 2009;72(3):224–31.

191. Tester DJ, Dura M, Carturan E, et al. A mechanism for sudden infant death syndrome (SIDS): stress-induced leak via ryanodine receptors. Heart Rhythm 2007;4(6):733–9.

192. van der Werf C, Hofman N, Tan HL, et al. Diagnostic yield in sudden unexplained death and aborted cardiac arrest in the young: the experience of a tertiary referral center in The Netherlands. Heart Rhythm 2010;7(10):1383–9.

193. Choi G, Kopplin LJ, Tester DJ, et al. Spectrum and frequency of cardiac channel defects in swimming-triggered arrhythmia syndromes. Circulation 2004; 110(15):2119–24.

194. Tester DJ, Medeiros-Domingo A, Will ML, et al. Unexplained drownings and the cardiac channelopathies: a molecular autopsy series. Mayo Clin Proc 2011;86(10):941–7.

195. Skinner JR, Crawford J, Smith W, et al. Prospective, population-based long QT molecular autopsy study of postmortem negative sudden death in 1 to 40 year olds. Heart Rhythm 2011; 8(3):412–9.

196. Behr ER, Dalageorgou C, Christiansen M, et al. Sudden arrhythmic death syndrome: familial evaluation identifies inheritable heart disease in the majority of families. Eur Heart J 2008;29(13): 1670–80.

197. Tan HL, Hofman N, van Langen IM, et al. Sudden unexplained death: heritability and diagnostic yield of cardiological and genetic examination in surviving relatives. Circulation 2005; 112(2):207–13.

198. Stone JR, Basso C, Baandrup UT, et al. Recommendations for processing cardiovascular surgical pathology specimens: a consensus statement from the Standards and Definitions Committee of the Society for Cardiovascular Pathology and the Association for European Cardiovascular Pathology. Cardiovasc Pathol 2012; 21(1):2–16.

Mechanisms Underlying Arrhythmogenesis in Long QT Syndrome

Charles Antzelevitch, PhD[a],*, Serge Sicouri, MD[b]

KEYWORDS
- QT interval • Electrophysiology • Arrhythmia
- Torsade de pointes • Sudden cardiac death

Prolongation of the QT interval, the time elapsed between ventricular depolarization and repolarization, on the surface electrocardiogram (ECG) is caused by an increase in the action potential duration (APD) of ventricular myocytes. It can result from several causes, including congenital defects that prolong APD, or can occur in response to an increasing number and diversity of drugs that prolong repolarization. Recent years have led to significant advances in our understanding of ion channelopathies associated with inherited cardiac arrhythmia syndromes responsible for the sudden death of infants, children, and young adults. Genetic variations giving rise to primary electrical diseases have been associated with long QT (LQTS), short QT (SQTS), Brugada (BrS), and early repolarization (ERS) syndromes, as well as catecholaminergic polymorphic ventricular tachycardia (VT). This article discusses the molecular, genetic, cellular, and ionic mechanisms underlying the development of arrhythmogenesis associated with LQTS.[1,2]

CHARACTERISTICS OF LONG QT SYNDROMES

The long QT syndromes are phenotypically and genotypically diverse, but have in common the appearance of long QT interval in the ECG, an atypical polymorphic VT known as torsade de pointes (TdP) and, in many but not all cases, a relatively high risk for sudden cardiac death.[3–5] A reduction in net repolarizing current secondary to a loss of function of outward ion channel currents or a gain of function of inward currents underlies the prolongation of the cardiac action potential and QT interval that attend both congenital and acquired forms of LQTS.[6,7]

Amplification of spatial dispersion of repolarization, secondary to an increase of transmural and transseptal dispersion of repolarization, is thought to underlie the development of the principal arrhythmogenic substrate. Early afterdepolarization (EAD)-induced triggered activity also contributes to the development of the substrate and provides the extrasystole that precipitates TdP arrhythmias observed under LQTS conditions (**Figs. 1** and **2**).[8,9] In vivo and in vitro models of LQTS have contributed to our understanding of the mechanisms involved in arrhythmogenesis. Models of the LQT1, LQT2, and LQT3 forms of the LQTS have been developed using the canine coronary-perfused left ventricular wedge preparation (see **Fig. 1**).[10] In these three forms of LQTS, preferential prolongation of the M-cell APD leads to an increase in both the QT interval and transmural dispersion of repolarization (TDR), the latter providing the substrate for the development of spontaneous and stimulation-induced TdP (**Fig. 3**).

Funding Sources: Supported by grants from the National Institutes of Health (HL 47678) and the Masons of New York State and Florida.

Disclosures: Dr Antzelevitch is a consultant for Gilead Sciences and AstraZeneca, and has received Research grant funds from Gilead Sciences, AstraZeneca, Merck, Cardiome, and Buchang Group.

[a] Masonic Medical Research Laboratory, 2150 Bleecker Street, Utica, NY 13501, USA

[b] Experimental Cardiology, Masonic Medical Research Laboratory, 2150 Bleecker Street, Utica, NY 13501, USA

* Corresponding author.

E-mail address: ca@mmrl.edu

Card Electrophysiol Clin 4 (2012) 17–27

doi:10.1016/j.ccep.2011.12.001

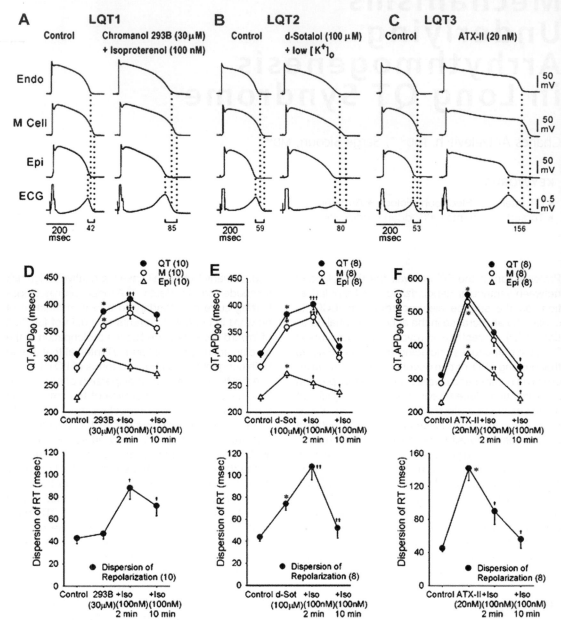

Fig. 1. Transmembrane action potentials (APs) and transmural electrocardiograms (ECGs) in control and LQT1 (*A*), LQT2 (*B*), and LQT3 (*C*) models of long QT syndrome (LQTS) (arterially perfused canine left ventricular wedge preparations). Isoproterenol + chromanol 293B (an I_{Ks} blocker), D-sotalol + low $[K^+]_o$, and ATX-II (an agent that slows inactivation of late I_{Na}) are used to mimic the LQT1, LQT2, and LQT3 syndromes, respectively. (*A–C*) Action potentials simultaneously recorded from endocardial (Endo), M, and epicardial (Epi) sites together with a transmural ECG. Basic cycle length = 2000 milliseconds. Transmural dispersion of repolarization (TDR) across the ventricular wall, defined as the difference in the repolarization time between M and Epi cells, is denoted below the ECG traces. (*D–F*) Effect of isoproterenol (Iso) in the LQT1, LQT2, and LQT3 models. In LQT1, Iso produces a persistent prolongation of the APD_{90} of the M cell and of the QT interval (at both 2 and 10 minutes), whereas the AP duration of 90 (APD_{90}) of the epicardial cell is always abbreviated, resulting in a persistent increase in TDR (*D*). In LQT2, Iso initially prolongs (2 minutes) and then abbreviates the QT interval and the APD_{90} of the M cell to the control level (10 minutes), whereas the APD_{90} of Epi cell is always abbreviated, resulting in a transient increase in TDR (*E*). In LQT3, Iso produced a persistent abbreviation of the QT interval and the APD_{90} of both M and Epi cells (at both 2 and 10 minutes), resulting in a persistent decrease in TDR (*F*). RT, repolarization time. *$P<.0005$ versus control; †$P<.0005$, ††$P<.005$, †††$P<.05$ versus 293B, D-sotalol (d-Sot), or ATX-II. (*Data from* Refs.[14–16])

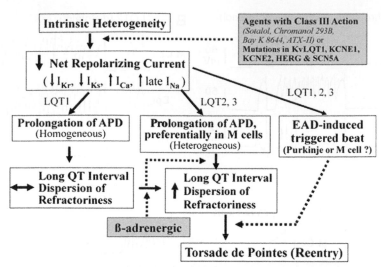

Fig. 2. Cellular and ionic mechanism underlying the development of torsade de pointes in the long QT syndrome. ADP, action-potential duration; EAD, early afterdepolarization. (*Adapted from* Antzelevitch C. The role of spatial dispersion of repolarization in inherited and acquired sudden cardiac death syndromes. Am J Physiol Heart Circ Physiol 2007;293:H2024–38; with permission.)

ARRHYTHMOGENIC MECHANISMS IN LQTS

The principal arrhythmogenic mechanism in LQTS relates to electrical heterogeneity and spatial dispersion of repolarization. Accentuation of spatial dispersion of refractoriness within the ventricular myocardium, secondary to exaggerated transmural or transseptal dispersion of repolarization, has been identified as the principal arrhythmogenic substrate in both acquired and congenital LQTS (see **Fig. 2**).[11,12] This exaggerated intrinsic heterogeneity, together with early and delayed afterdepolarization (EAD and DAD)-induced triggered activity, both caused by reduction in net repolarizing current, underlies the substrate and trigger for the development of TdP arrhythmias observed under LQTS conditions (see **Fig. 3**).[9,13] Preferential prolongation of the M-cell APD leads to an increase in the QT interval and an increase in TDR, which contributes to the development of spontaneous as well as stimulation-induced TdP (see **Fig. 2**).[12,14–18] The spatial dispersion of repolarization is further exaggerated by sympathetic influences in congenital LQT1 and LQT2, accounting for the great sensitivity of patients with these genotypes to adrenergic stimuli.

CONGENITAL LQTS

Congenital LQTS is subdivided into distinct genotypes distinguished by mutations in at least 13 different ion-channel and structural anchoring genes located on chromosomes 3, 4, 6, 7, 11, 17, and 21 (**Table 1**).[19–27] Two patterns of inheritance have been identified: (1) a rare autosomal recessive disease associated with deafness (Jervell and Lange-Nielsen), caused by 2 genes that encode for the slowly activating delayed rectifier potassium channel (KCNQ1 and KCNE1), and (2) a much more common autosomal dominant form known as the Romano-Ward syndrome, caused by mutations in 13 different genes (see **Table 1**). Seven of the 13 genes encode for cardiac potassium channels, causing a loss of function in outward current carried by these channels. Five of the genes encode for proteins that when mutated lead to an increase in late I_{Na} or I_{Ca}. One of the genes encodes for a protein called ankyrin B (*ANKB*), which is involved in the anchoring of ion channels to the cellular membrane.

The prevalence of this disorder is estimated at 1 to 2 per 10,000. The ECG diagnosis is based on the presence of prolonged repolarization (QT interval) and abnormal T-wave morphology.[28] In the different genotypes, cardiac events may be precipitated by physical or emotional stress (LQT1) or a startle (LQT2), or may occur at rest or during sleep (LQT3). Anti-adrenergic intervention with β-blockers is the mainstay of therapy. For patients unresponsive to this approach, a late sodium channel blocker, an implantable cardioverter-defibrillator, and/or cardiac sympathetic denervation may be therapeutic alternatives.[29–34]

LQT1

LQT1, the most prevalent of the congenital LQTS,[35] is caused by a loss of function of the slowly activating delayed rectifier potassium current (I_{Ks}). Inhibition of I_{Ks} using chromanol 293B has been

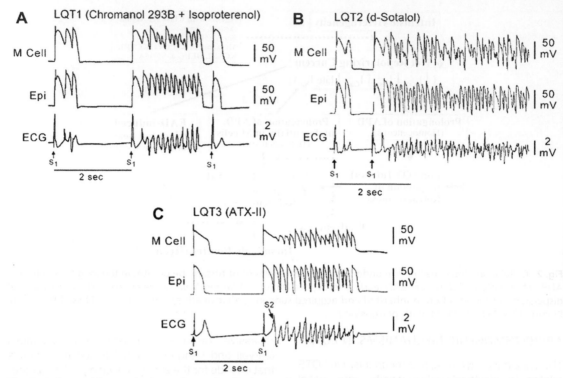

Fig. 3. Polymorphic ventricular tachycardia displaying features of torsade de pointes (TdP) in the long QT 1 (LQT1) (*A*), LQT2 (*B*), and LQT3 (*C*) models (arterially perfused canine left ventricular wedge preparations). Isoproterenol + chromanol 293B, D-sotalol, and ATX-II are used to mimic the 3 long QT syndromes (LQTs), respectively. Each trace shows action potentials simultaneously recorded from M and epicardial (Epi) cells together with a transmural electrocardiogram. The preparation was paced from the endocardial surface at a basic cycle length of 2000 milliseconds (S1). (*A, B*) Spontaneous TdP induced in the LQT1 and LQT2 models, respectively. In both models, the first groupings show spontaneous ventricular premature beat (or couplets) that fail to induce TdP, and a second grouping that shows spontaneous premature beats that succeed. The premature response appears to originate in the deep subendocardium (M or Purkinje). (*C*) Programmed electrical stimulation-induced TdP in the LQT3 model. ATX-II produced very significant dispersion of repolarization (first grouping). A single extrastimulus (S2) applied to the epicardial surface at an S1-S2 interval of 320 milliseconds initiates TdP (second grouping). (*Adapted from* Refs.[14–16])

shown to lead to uniform prolongation of APD in all 3 cell types in the wedge, causing little change in TDR (see **Fig. 1**). Although the QT interval is prolonged, TdP does not occur under these conditions, nor can it be induced. The addition of isoproterenol results in abbreviation of epicardial and endocardial APD, whereas the M-cell APD either prolongs or remains the same. The dramatic increase in TDR provides the substrate for the development of spontaneous as well as stimulation-induced TdP (**Fig. 4**).[14] These results support the thesis that the problem with the LQTS is not the long QT interval, but rather the increase in TDR that often accompanies the prolongation of the QT interval. The combination of I_{Ks} block and β-adrenergic stimulation creates a broad-based T wave in the perfused wedge, similar to that observed in patients with LQT1. These findings provide us with an understanding of the sensitivity of patients with LQT1 to sympathetic influences (see **Fig. 1**A, D).[3,36]

LQT2

The second most prevalent form of congenital LQTS, LQT2, is caused by a loss of function of the rapidly activating delayed rectifier potassium current (I_{Kr}). I_{Kr} inhibition is also responsible for most cases of acquired LQTS. In the wedge, inhibition of I_{Kr} with D-sotalol produces a preferential prolongation of the M cells, resulting in accentuation of TDR and spontaneous as well as stimulation-induced TdP (see **Fig. 2**). When I_{Kr} block is combined with hypokalemia, bifurcated T waves develop in the wedge preparation, similar to those seen in patients with LQT2. Isoproterenol further exaggerates TDR and increases the incidence of TdP in this model, but only transiently (see **Fig. 1**B, E).

Table 1
Congenital long QT syndrome (LQTS)

		Rhythm	Inheritance	Locus	Ion Channel	Gene
LQTS	(RW)	TdP	AD			
	LQT1			11p15	$\downarrow I_{Ks}$	KCNQ1, KvLQT1
	LQT2			7q35	$\downarrow I_{Kr}$	KCNH2, HERG
	LQT3			3p21	$\uparrow I_{Na}$	SCN5A, Na$_v$1.5
	LQT4			4q25		ANKB, ANK2
	LQT5			21q22	$\downarrow I_{Ks}$	KCNE1, minK
	LQT6			21q22	$\downarrow I_{Kr}$	KCNE2, MiRP1
	LQT7	(Andersen-Tawil syndrome)		17q23	$\downarrow I_{K1}$	KCNJ2, Kir 2.1
	LQT8	(Timothy syndrome)		6q8A	$\uparrow I_{Ca}$	CACNA1C, Ca$_v$1.2
	LQT9			3p25	$\uparrow I_{Na}$	CAV3, Caveolin-3
	LQT10			11q23.3	$\uparrow I_{Na}$	SCN4B. Na$_v$β4
	LQT11			7q21-q22	$\downarrow I_{Ks}$	AKAP9, Yotiao
	LQT12			20q11.2	$\uparrow I_{Na}$	SNTA1, α-1 Syntrophin
	LQT13			11q24 1	$\downarrow I_{K-ACh}$	KCNJ5, Kir3.4
LQTS (JLN)		TdP	AR	11p15	$\downarrow\downarrow I_{Ks}$	KCNQ1, KvLQT1
				21q22	$\downarrow\downarrow I_{Ks}$	KCNE1, minK

Abbreviations: ACh, acetylcholine; AD, autosomal dominant; AR, autosomal recessive; BrS, Brugada syndrome; CPVT, catecholaminergic polymorphic ventricular tachycardia; JLN, Jervell and Lange-Nielsen.

LQT3

LQT3, encountered in approximately 8% of genotyped probands, is caused by a gain of function of late sodium current (late I_{Na}). Augmentation of late I_{Na} using the sea anemone toxin ATX-II produces a preferential prolongation of the M-cell action potential in the wedge, resulting in a marked increase in TDR and development of TdP (see **Fig. 2**). Because epicardial APD is also significantly prolonged, there is delay in the onset of the T wave in the wedge, as observed in the clinical syndrome.[15] Under these conditions, β-adrenergic stimulation abbreviates APD of all cell types, reducing TDR and preventing or suppressing TdP (see **Fig. 1C, F**).[16]

Sympathetic activation displays a very different time course in the case of LQT1 and LQT2, both in experimental models (see **Fig. 1**) and in the clinic.[9,37] In LQT1, isoproterenol produces an increase in TDR that is most prominent during the first 2 minutes, but which persists, although to a lesser extent, during steady state. TdP incidence is enhanced during the initial period as well as during steady state. In LQT2, isoproterenol produces only a transient increase in TDR that persists for less than 2 minutes. TdP incidence is therefore enhanced only for a brief period of time. These differences in time course may explain the important differences in autonomic activity and other gene-specific triggers that contribute to events in patients with different LQTS genotypes.[35,36]

Although β-blockers are considered the first-line therapy for patients with LQTS, there is no clear evidence that they are of benefit in LQT3. Experimental and recent clinical data suggest that patients with LQT3 might benefit from Na$^+$ channel blockers, such as mexiletine, flecainide, and ranolazine.[29–34,38,39] Experimental data have shown that mexiletine reduces transmural dispersion and prevents TdP in LQT3 as well as LQT1 and LQT2, suggesting that agents that block the late sodium current may be effective in all forms of LQTS.[14,15] The late I_{Na} blocker ranolazine is effective in abbreviating QT interval and suppressing TdP in experimental models of LQT3[40–42] and in significantly abbreviating QT$_c$ in patients with LQT3.[31]

LQT7

Andersen-Tawil syndrome (ATS1), also known as LQT7, is a clinical disorder consisting of potassium-sensitive periodic paralysis, prolonged QT intervals, ventricular arrhythmias, and dysmorphic features, caused by mutations in the KCNJ2 gene, which encodes the Kir2.1 that forms the I_{K1} channel.[43,44] An experimental model of this syndrome has been developed and characterized.[45] Inhibition of I_{K1} using BaCl$_2$ (10–30 μM) produced a homogeneous prolongation of APD of the 3 cell types, thus prolonging QT interval without an increase in TDR. Low extracellular potassium (2.0 mM) and isoproterenol (20–50 nM)

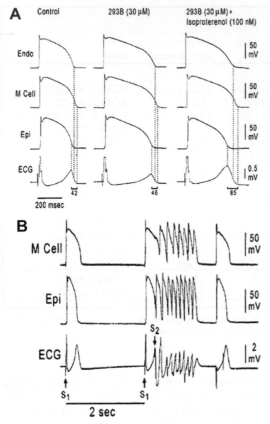

Fig. 4. Experimental model of LQT1-induced torsade de pointes (TdP) in the wedge preparation. (*A*) From top to bottom: endocardial (Endo), M, and epicardial (Epi) action potentials and an electrocardiogram (ECG). From left to right: control conditions, effect of chromanol 293B (30 μM), and effect of addition of isoproterenol (100 nM) to the perfusate. Left ventricle wedge preparation; basic cycle length = 2000 milliseconds. Transmural dispersion of repolarization and T_{peak}-T_{end} increased from 42 (control) to 46 (chromanol 293B) to 85 milliseconds (chromanol 293B + isoproterenol). A single extrastimulus (S2) applied to the Epi surface (S1-S2 interval = 320 milliseconds) initiated TdP (*B*). (*Adapted from* Refs.[14–16])

in the continued presence of 10 μM BaCl$_2$ did not significantly increase TDR but increased ectopic extrasystolic activity due to enhanced automaticity in the Purkinje system of the ventricle. Spontaneous TdP arrhythmias were never observed, nor could they be induced with programmed electrical stimulation under any of the conditions studied. These results are consistent with the clinical presentation of ATS1, which is associated with a great deal of ectopy but rarely with TdP. The study provides further support for the hypothesis that the increase in TDR, rather than the QT interval, is responsible for development of TdP.

LQT8

Timothy syndrome, also known as LQT8, is a multisystem disease secondary to mutations in the calcium channel Ca$_v$1.2 encoded by *CACNA1c*. Because the calcium channel Ca$_v$1.2 is present in many tissues, patients with Timothy syndrome have many clinical manifestations including congenital heart disease, autism, syndactyly, and immune deficiency.[46,47] An experimental model of this syndrome has been developed.[48]

Mutations in 10 other genes have been associated with LQTS in recent years (see **Table 1**). These genetic variations, which include structural proteins as well as other ion channel proteins, are relatively rare.

Genotype-phenotype correlation studies have demonstrated that significant differences exist among patients with LQT1, LQT2, and LQT3 forms of LQTS; these 3 forms account for 95% of all genotyped patients. Gene-specific ECG patterns have been identified (see **Fig. 1**),[49,50] and the trigger for cardiac events has been shown to be gene specific.[35] Patients with LQT1 experience 97% of cardiac events during physical activity as opposed to those with LQT3, who present most cardiac events at rest or during sleep. Auditory stimuli and arousal have been identified as relatively specific triggers for patients with LQT2, whereas swimming has been identified as a predisposing setting for cardiac events in patients with LQT1.[51,52]

Table 2	
Drugs withdrawn from the market due to QT liability	
Drug (Clinical Use)	**Year Withdrawn**
Prenylamine (antianginal)	1988
Lidoflazine (antianginal)	1989
Terodiline (urinary incontinence)	1991
Sertindole[a] (antipsychotic)	1998
Terfenadine (antihistamine)	1998
Astemizole (antihistamine)	1999
Grepafloxacin (antibiotic)	1999
Cisapride (gastric prokinetic)	2000
Levacetylmethadol (methadone substitution)	2001
Droperidol (tranquillizer/ analgesic)	2001
Thioridazine (antipsychotic)	2005
Clobutinol (antitussive)	2007
Propoxyphene (analgesic)	2009

[a] Reintroduced in 2005 after reassessment of risk-benefit.

Table 3
Drugs that block I_{Kr} and/or I_{Ks}, prolong the QT interval or induce torsade de pointes (TdP), and their ability to induce early afterdepolarizations (EADs) and increase dispersion of ventricular repolarization[a]

Drug[b]	Blocks I_{Kr}/I_{Ks}	Prolongs QT_c Interval	TdP Reported	Induces EADs	Increases Dispersion of Repolarization[c]
Antiarrhythmics					
Almokalant	+	+	+	+	+
Amiodarone	+	+	+	−	±
Azimilide	+	+	+	+	+
Dofetilide	+	+	+	+	+
Ibutilide	+	+	+	+	+
Quinidine	+	+	+	+	+
Sotalol	+	+	+	+	+
Antihistamines					
Astemizole	+	+	+	+	+
Terfenadine	+	+	+	+	+
Antibiotics					
Erythromycin	+	+	+	+	+
Calcium Channel Antagonists					
Diltiazem	+	±	−	−	−
Verapamil	+	±	−	−	−
Mibefradil	+	+	+	+	−
Bepridil	+	+	+	+	+
Psychotherapeutic					
Sertindole	+	+	+	−	−
Droperidol	+	+	+	+	?
Miscellaneous					
Cisapride	+	+	+	+	+
Sodium pentobarbital	+	+	−	−	−
Ketanserin	+	+	+	+	+
Ranolazine	+	+	−	−	−

Abbreviations: +, response to drug noted; −, lack of response to drug noted; ±, response noted in some studies but not others; ?, data not found.

[a] Includes drugs known to inhibit the rapidly activating delayed rectifier potassium channel (I_{Kr}) and slowly activating delayed rectifier potassium channel (I_{Ks}), prolong QT or induce TdP, for which data are available relative to their actions to cause EADs or increase dispersion of ventricular repolarization.

[b] Based on a review of the literature of QT-prolonging drugs reported to inhibit I_{Kr} and/or I_{Ks}. Data are derived from humans, nonclinical models, or both. Nonclinical models include anesthetized animals, isolated hearts, and multicellular and single cardiac-cell preparations.

[c] Dispersion of repolarization includes both QT dispersion (ie, interlead variability of QT interval in humans) and/or transmural and interventricular dispersion of repolarization (ie, differences in action potential duration) in nonclinical models.

Adapted from Belardinelli L, Antzelevitch C, Vos MA. Assessing predictors of drug-induced torsade de pointes. Trends Pharmacol Sci 2003;24:621; with permission.

Priori and colleagues[53] proposed the first risk stratification scheme based on genotype in 2003. QT interval, genotype, and gender were all significantly associated with events. A QT_c interval of greater than 500 milliseconds in LQT2 or LQT3 forecasts a worse prognosis. In 2004 the same investigators reported that the response to β-blockers is also genotype specific, with patients with LQT1 showing greater protection in response to β-blockers than patients with LQT2 or LQT3.[54]

Patients with LQT2 harboring pore mutations show a more severe clinical course and experience a higher frequency of arrhythmia-related cardiac events, occurring at an earlier age than for subjects with nonpore mutations.[55] KCNH2 missense mutations located in the transmembrane S5-loop-S6 region were again shown to be associated with the greatest risk in a recent study.[56]

ACQUIRED LQTS

Acquired LQTS refers to a syndrome similar to the congenital form, but which is attributable to environmental factors or exposure to drugs that prolong the duration of the ventricular AP.[57] A prolonged APD can be caused by drug effects on a single or many ion channels, pumps, or exchangers. Inhibition of the I_{Kr} is the most common cause of drug-induced QT prolongation.[57] Many drugs that block I_{Kr}, including agents such as quinidine, amiodarone, and azimilide, also inhibit the I_{Ks}. Some drugs and toxins, including DPI 201-106, anthopleurin-A, and ATX-II,[58–60] prolong the QT interval by augmenting late I_{Na}. Many drugs block multiple cardiac ion channels, thus causing a more complex alteration in the morphology of action potential.

I_{Kr} block and QT prolongation have attracted attention in recent years because of their association with life-threatening cardiac arrhythmias, such as TdP.[6,13,61–63] Thirteen drugs have been withdrawn from the market worldwide in the past decade because of this potential arrhythmogenic syndrome (**Table 2**). Antiarrhythmic drugs with class III action capable of prolonging cardiac repolarization by blocking potassium channels were among the first to be linked to TdP arrhythmia. Syncope arising after the initiation of quinidine therapy has been recognized for more than 80 years.[64] The incidence of TdP in patients treated with quinidine is estimated to range between 2.0% and 8.8%.[64–66] DL-Sotalol has been associated with an incidence ranging from 1.8% to 4.8%.[67–69] A similar incidence has been described for newer class III agents, such as dofetilide[70] and ibutilide.[71] An ever-increasing number and variety of noncardiovascular agents, most acting via inhibition of I_{Kr}, have also been shown to aggravate and/or precipitate TdP.[6,61] More than 50 commercially available or investigational noncardiovascular and 20 cardiovascular nonantiarrhythmic drugs have been implicated. **Table 3** summarizes the different drugs known to induce acquired forms of LQTS, and their ability to induce EADs and increase dispersion of ventricular repolarization, thus generating the trigger and substrate for development of TdP.

Other forms of acquired long QT have been recognized, including the QT prolongation that accompanies hypertrophic cardiomyopathy, dilated cardiomyopathy, or heart failure, and the QT prolongation occurring in the early phases after myocardial infarction, as well as exaggerated QT prolongation associated with bradycardia or electrolyte imbalance.[72–76]

REFERENCES

1. Kaufman ES. Mechanisms and clinical management of inherited channelopathies: long QT syndrome, Brugada syndrome, catecholaminergic polymorphic ventricular tachycardia, and short QT syndrome. Heart Rhythm 2009;6:S51–5.
2. Antzelevitch C. The role of spatial dispersion of repolarization in inherited and acquired sudden cardiac death syndromes. Am J Physiol Heart Circ Physiol 2007;293:H2024–38.
3. Schwartz PJ. The idiopathic long QT syndrome: progress and questions. Am Heart J 1985;109:399–411.
4. Moss AJ, Schwartz PJ, Crampton RS, et al. The long QT syndrome: prospective longitudinal study of 328 families. Circulation 1991;84:1136–44.
5. Zipes DP. The long QT interval syndrome. A Rosetta stone for sympathetic related ventricular tachyarrhythmias. Circulation 1991;84:1414–9.
6. Roden DM. Drug-induced prolongation of the QT interval. N Engl J Med 2004;350:1013–22.
7. Dumaine R, Antzelevitch C. Molecular mechanisms underlying the long QT syndrome. Curr Opin Cardiol 2002;17:36–42.
8. Antzelevitch C. Heterogeneity of cellular repolarization in LQTS: the role of M cells. Eur Heart J Suppl 2001;3:K2–16.
9. Antzelevitch C, Shimizu W. Cellular mechanisms underlying the long QT syndrome. Curr Opin Cardiol 2002;17:43–51.
10. Shimizu W, Antzelevitch C. Effects of a K^+ channel opener to reduce transmural dispersion of repolarization and prevent torsade de pointes in LQT1, LQT2, and LQT3 models of the long-QT syndrome. Circulation 2000;102:706–12.
11. Antzelevitch C. Heterogeneity and cardiac arrhythmias: an overview. Heart Rhythm 2007;4:964–72.
12. Sicouri S, Glass A, Ferreiro M, et al. Transseptal dispersion of repolarization and its role in the development of torsade de pointes arrhythmias. J Cardiovasc Electrophysiol 2010;21:441–7.
13. Belardinelli L, Antzelevitch C, Vos MA. Assessing predictors of drug-induced torsade de pointes. Trends Pharmacol Sci 2003;24:619–25.
14. Shimizu W, Antzelevitch C. Cellular basis for the ECG features of the LQT1 form of the long QT syndrome: effects of b-adrenergic agonists and antagonists and sodium channel blockers on

transmural dispersion of repolarization and torsade de pointes. Circulation 1998;98:2314–22.

15. Shimizu W, Antzelevitch C. Sodium channel block with mexiletine is effective in reducing dispersion of repolarization and preventing torsade de pointes in LQT2 and LQT3 models of the long-QT syndrome. Circulation 1997;96:2038–47.

16. Shimizu W, Antzelevitch C. Differential effects of beta-adrenergic agonists and antagonists in LQT1, LQT2 and LQT3 models of the long QT syndrome. J Am Coll Cardiol 2000;35:778–86.

17. Ueda N, Zipes DP, Wu J. Prior ischemia enhances arrhythmogenicity in isolated canine ventricular wedge model of long QT 3. Cardiovasc Res 2004; 63:69–76.

18. Ueda N, Zipes DP, Wu J. Functional and transmural modulation of M cell behavior in canine ventricular wall. Am J Physiol Heart Circ Physiol 2004;287: H2569–75.

19. Wang Q, Shen J, Splawski I, et al. SCN5A mutations associated with an inherited cardiac arrhythmia, long QT syndrome. Cell 1995;80:805–11.

20. Mohler PJ, Schott JJ, Gramolini AO, et al. Ankyrin-B mutation causes type 4 long-QT cardiac arrhythmia and sudden cardiac death. Nature 2003;421:634–9.

21. Plaster NM, Tawil R, Tristani-Firouzi M, et al. Mutations in Kir2.1 cause the developmental and episodic electrical phenotypes of Andersen's syndrome. Cell 2001;105:511–9.

22. Curran ME, Splawski I, Timothy KW, et al. A molecular basis for cardiac arrhythmia: HERG mutations cause long QT syndrome. Cell 1995;80:795–803.

23. Wang Q, Curran ME, Splawski I, et al. Positional cloning of a novel potassium channel gene: KVLQT1 mutations cause cardiac arrhythmias. Nat Genet 1996;12:17–23.

24. Splawski I, Tristani-Firouzi M, Lehmann MH, et al. Mutations in the hminK gene cause long QT syndrome and suppress I_{Ks} function. Nat Genet 1997;17:338–40.

25. Medeiros-Domingo A, Kaku T, Tester DJ, et al. SCN4B-encoded sodium channel b4 subunit in congenital long-QT syndrome. Circulation 2007; 116:134–42.

26. Vatta M, Ackerman MJ, Ye B, et al. Mutant caveolin-3 induces persistent late sodium current and is associated with long-QT syndrome. Circulation 2006; 114:2104–12.

27. Yang Y, Yang Y, Liang B, et al. Identification of a Kir3.4 mutation in congenital long QT syndrome. Am J Hum Genet 2010;86:872–80.

28. Schwartz PJ, Priori SG, Napolitano C. The long QT syndrome. In: Zipes DP, Jalife J, editors. Cardiac electrophysiology: from cell to bedside. 3rd edition. Philadelphia: WB Saunders; 2000. p. 597–615.

29. Moss AJ, Zareba W, Hall WJ, et al. Effectiveness and limitations of beta-blocker therapy in congenital long-QT syndrome. Circulation 2000;101:616–23.

30. Schwartz PJ, Priori SG, Cerrone M, et al. Left cardiac sympathetic denervation in the management of high-risk patients affected by the long-QT syndrome. Circulation 2004;109:1826–33.

31. Moss AJ, Zareba W, Schwarz KQ, et al. Ranolazine shortens repolarization in patients with sustained inward sodium current due to type-3 long-QT syndrome. J Cardiovasc Electrophysiol 2008;19:1289–93.

32. Shimizu W, Aiba T, Antzelevitch C. Specific therapy based on the genotype and cellular mechanism in inherited cardiac arrhythmias. Long QT syndrome and Brugada syndrome. Curr Pharm Des 2005;11:1561–72.

33. Napolitano C, Bloise R, Priori SG. Gene-specific therapy for inherited arrhythmogenic diseases. Pharmacol Ther 2006;110:1–13.

34. Antzelevitch C, Burashnikov A, Sicouri S, et al. Electrophysiological basis for the antiarrhythmic actions of ranolazine. Heart Rhythm 2011;8:1281–90.

35. Schwartz PJ, Priori SG, Spazzolini C, et al. Genotype-phenotype correlation in the long-QT syndrome: gene-specific triggers for life-threatening arrhythmias. Circulation 2001;103:89–95.

36. Ali RH, Zareba W, Moss A, et al. Clinical and genetic variables associated with acute arousal and nonarousal-related cardiac events among subjects with long QT syndrome. Am J Cardiol 2000;85:457–61.

37. Noda T, Takaki H, Kurita T, et al. Gene-specific response of dynamic ventricular repolarization to sympathetic stimulation in LQT1, LQT2 and LQT3 forms of congenital long QT syndrome. Eur Heart J 2002;23:975–83.

38. Windle JR, Geletka RC, Moss AJ, et al. Normalization of ventricular repolarization with flecainide in long QT syndrome patients with SCN5A: deltaKPQ mutation. Ann Noninvasive Electrocardiol 2001;6:153–8.

39. Roden DM. Pharmacogenetics and drug-induced arrhythmias. Cardiovasc Res 2001;50:224–31.

40. Antzelevitch C, Belardinelli L, Zygmunt AC, et al. Electrophysiologic effects of ranolazine: a novel anti-anginal agent with antiarrhythmic properties. Circulation 2004;110:904–10.

41. Antzelevitch C, Belardinelli L, Wu L, et al. Electrophysiologic properties and antiarrhythmic actions of a novel anti-anginal agent. J Cardiovasc Pharmacol Ther 2004;9(Suppl 1):S65–83.

42. Wu L, Shryock JC, Song Y, et al. Antiarrhythmic effects of ranolazine in a guinea pig in vitro model of long-QT syndrome. J Pharmacol Exp Ther 2004; 310:599–605.

43. Tristani-Firouzi M, Jensen JL, Donaldson MR, et al. Functional and clinical characterization of KCNJ2 mutations associated with LQT7 (Andersen syndrome). J Clin Invest 2002;110:381–8.

44. Andelfinger G, Tapper AR, Welch RC, et al. KCNJ2 mutation results in Andersen syndrome with sex-specific cardiac and skeletal muscle phenotypes. Am J Hum Genet 2002;71:663–8.

45. Tsuboi M, Antzelevitch C. Cellular basis for electrocardiographic and arrhythmic manifestations of Andersen-Tawil syndrome (LQT7). Heart Rhythm 2006;3:328–35.

46. Splawski I, Timothy KW, Sharpe LM, et al. Ca$_v$1.2 calcium channel dysfunction causes a multisystem disorder including arrhythmia and autism. Cell 2004;119:19–31.

47. Splawski I, Timothy KW, Decher N, et al. Severe arrhythmia disorder caused by cardiac L-type calcium channel mutations. Proc Natl Acad Sci U S A 2005;102:8089–96.

48. Sicouri S, Timothy KW, Zygmunt AC, et al. Cellular basis for the electrocardiographic and arrhythmic manifestations of Timothy syndrome: effects of ranolazine. Heart Rhythm 2007;4:638–47.

49. Moss AJ, Zareba W, Benhorin J, et al. ECG T-wave patterns in genetically distinct forms of the hereditary long QT syndrome. Circulation 1995;92:2929–34.

50. Zhang L, Timothy KW, Vincent GM, et al. Spectrum of ST-T-wave patterns and repolarization parameters in congenital long-QT syndrome: ECG findings identify genotypes. Circulation 2000;102:2849–55.

51. Moss AJ, Robinson JL, Gessman L, et al. Comparison of clinical and genetic variables of cardiac events associated with loud noise versus swimming among subjects with the long QT syndrome. Am J Cardiol 1999;84:876–9.

52. Ackerman MJ, Tester DJ, Porter CJ. Swimming, a gene-specific arrhythmogenic trigger for inherited long QT syndrome. Mayo Clin Proc 1999;74:1088–94.

53. Priori SG, Schwartz PJ, Napolitano C, et al. Risk stratification in the long-QT syndrome. N Engl J Med 2003;348:1866–74.

54. Priori SG, Napolitano C, Schwartz PJ, et al. Association of long QT syndrome loci and cardiac events among patients treated with beta-blockers. JAMA 2004;292:1341–4.

55. Moss AJ, Zareba W, Kaufman ES, et al. Increased risk of arrhythmic events in long-QT syndrome with mutations in the pore region of the human *ether-a-go-go*-related gene potassium channel. Circulation 2002;105:794–9.

56. Shimizu W, Moss AJ, Wilde AA, et al. Genotype-phenotype aspects of type 2 long QT syndrome. J Am Coll Cardiol 2009;54:2052–62.

57. Bednar MM, Harrigan EP, Anziano RJ, et al. The QT interval. Prog Cardiovasc Dis 2001;43:1–45.

58. Gwathmey JK, Slawsky MT, Briggs GM, et al. Role of intracellular sodium in the regulation of intracellular calcium and contractility. Effects of DPI 201-106 on excitation-contraction coupling in human ventricular myocardium. J Clin Invest 1988;82:1592–605.

59. Li CZ, Wang HW, Liu JL, et al. Effect of ATXII on opening modes of myocyte sodium channel, action potential and QT intervals of ECG. Sheng Li Xue Bao 2001;53:111–6 [in Chinese].

60. Hanck DA, Sheets MF. Modification of inactivation in cardiac sodium channels: ionic current studies with anthopleurin-A toxin. J Gen Physiol 1995;106:601–16.

61. Fenichel RR, Malik M, Antzelevitch C, et al. Drug-induced torsade de pointes and implications for drug development. J Cardiovasc Electrophysiol 2004;15:475–95.

62. Antzelevitch C, El-Sherif N, Rosenbaum D, et al. Cellular mechanisms underlying the long QT syndrome. J Cardiovasc Electrophysiol 2003;14:114–5.

63. Haverkamp W, Breithardt G, Camm AJ, et al. The potential for QT prolongation and proarrhythmia by non-antiarrhythmic drugs: clinical and regulatory implications. Report on a Policy Conference of the European Society of Cardiology. Cardiovasc Res 2000;47:219–33.

64. Selzer A, Wray HW. Quinidine syncope. Paroxysmal ventricular fibrillation occurring during treatment of chronic atrial arrhythmias. Circulation 1964;30:17–26.

65. Roden DM, Woosley RL, Primm RK. Incidence and clinical features of the quinidine-associated long-QT syndrome: implications for patient care. Am Heart J 1986;111:1088–93.

66. Kay GN, Plumb VJ, Arciniegas JG, et al. Torsade de pointes: the long-short initiating sequence and other clinical features: observations in 32 patients. J Am Coll Cardiol 1983;2:806–17.

67. Haverkamp W, Martinez-Rubio A, Hief C, et al. Efficacy and safety of d,l-sotalol in patients with ventricular tachycardia and in survivors of cardiac arrest. J Am Coll Cardiol 1997;30:487–95.

68. Lehmann MH, Hardy S, Archibald D, et al. Sex difference in risk of torsade de pointes with d,l-sotalol. Circulation 1996;94:2535–41.

69. Hohnloser SH. Proarrhythmia with class III antiarrhythmic drugs: types, risks, and management. Am J Cardiol 1997;80:82G–9G.

70. Kober L, Bloch Thomsen PE, Moller M, et al. Effect of dofetilide in patients with recent myocardial infarction and left-ventricular dysfunction: a randomised trial. Lancet 2000;356:2052–8.

71. Stambler BS, Wood MA, Ellenbogen KA, et al. Efficacy and safety of repeated intravenous doses of ibutilide for rapid conversion of atrial flutter or fibrillation. Ibutilide Repeat Dose Study Investigators. Circulation 1996;94:1613–21.

72. Tomaselli GF, Marban E. Electrophysiological remodeling in hypertrophy and heart failure. Cardiovasc Res 1999;42:270–83.

73. Sipido KR, Volders PG, De Groot SH, et al. Enhanced Ca^{2+} release and Na/Ca exchange activity in

hypertrophied canine ventricular myocytes: potential link between contractile adaptation and arrhythmogenesis. Circulation 2000;102:2137–44.

74. Volders PG, Sipido KR, Vos MA, et al. Downregulation of delayed rectifier K(+) currents in dogs with chronic complete atrioventricular block and acquired torsades de pointes. Circulation 1999;100:2455–61.

75. Undrovinas AI, Maltsev VA, Sabbah HN. Repolarization abnormalities in cardiomyocytes of dogs with chronic heart failure: role of sustained inward current. Cell Mol Life Sci 1999;55:494–505.

76. Maltsev VA, Sabbah HN, Higgins RS, et al. Novel, ultraslow inactivating sodium current in human ventricular cardiomyocytes. Circulation 1998;98:2545–52.

Diagnostic Evaluation of Long QT Syndrome

Wataru Shimizu, MD, PhD

KEYWORDS

- Long QT syndrome • Provocative testing
- Torsades de pointes • Holter recording

Congenital long QT syndrome (LQTS) is one of the heritable channelopathies, characterized by prolongation of QT interval in the standard 12-lead electrocardiogram (ECG) and a polymorphic ventricular tachycardia known as torsades de pointes (TdP) often observed in a situation of sympathetic stimulation.[1] The clinical diagnosis of congenital LQTS is based mainly on the rate-corrected QT (QTc) interval at rest, cardiac events such as syncope, aborted cardiac arrest and sudden cardiac death, and a family history of apparent LQTS.[2] The electrocardiographic diagnosis at baseline, however, misses some patients affected by congenital LQTS (so-called concealed LQTS) as evidenced by syncopal events occurring among family members with a normal QT interval.[3] An estimated 30% to 40% of genetically affected subjects have concealed LQTS with a normal or borderline QTc interval at rest in congenital LQTS. Many but not all patients with congenital LQTS suffer from cardiac events such as syncope and/or sudden cardiac death during physical exercise or mental stress. Therefore, provocative testing using catecholamine infusion or exercise was long used to unmask concealed forms of congenital LQTS, before genetic testing became available.[4] The first 2 genes responsible for LQTS (LQT1 and LQT2) were identified in 1995. Since then, molecular genetic studies have revealed a total of 13 genetic subtypes of congenital LQTS caused predominantly by cardiac-channel mutations or mutations involving key β or auxiliary subunits.[5–9] Among the 13 genetic subtypes, LQT1, LQT2, and LQT3 comprise the vast majority

of genotyped LQTS and approximately 75% of all LQTS.[10] In this article, the role of provocative testing, including catecholamine provocative testing, exercise stress testing, and so forth, in the evaluation of congenital LQTS, specifically diagnosing (unmasking) concealed LQTS and predicting genotypes of LQTS (LQT1, LQT2, and LQT3), is reviewed.

LOW PENETRANCE OF CONGENITAL LQTS

Concealed or low-penetrance LQTS was genetically proved for the first time by Vincent and colleagues,[11] who reported that 5 (6%) of 82 mutation carriers from 3 LQT1 families had a normal QT interval. Priori and colleagues[12] conducted molecular screening in 9 families with apparently sporadic cases of LQTS, and demonstrated a very low penetrance (38%, 9 of 24 patients). Swan and colleagues[13] reported that the sensitivity and specificity for identifying genotype-positive patients were 53% and 100%, respectively, in an LQT1 family with a specific KCNQ1 mutation (D188 N). Priori and colleagues[14] also showed, in more recent larger study of genotyped LQTS, that the percentage of genetically affected patients with a normal QTc interval was significantly higher in the LQT1 (36%) than in the LQT2 (19%) or the LQT3 (10%) syndromes. These findings strongly suggest the need for novel tools to unveil concealed mutation carriers of LQTS, especially those with LQT1. The identification of patients with concealed LQTS affords the opportunity to initiate potentially life-saving pharmacotherapies as well as health care and lifestyle modifications.

Dr Shimizu was supported in part by the Research Grant for the Cardiovascular Diseases (21C-8, 22-4-7, H23-114) from the Ministry of Health, Labor and Welfare, Japan, and Grant-in-Aid for Scientific Research on Innovative Areas (22136011).

Division of Arrhythmia and Electrophysiology, Department of Cardiovascular Medicine, National Cerebral and Cardiovascular Center, 5-7-1 Fujishiro-dai, Suita, Osaka, 565-8565 Japan
E-mail address: wshimizu@hsp.ncvc.go.jp

Card Electrophysiol Clin 4 (2012) 29–37
doi:10.1016/j.ccep.2011.12.005

cardiacEP.theclinics.com

EPINEPHRINE PROVOCATIVE TESTING

Intravenous infusion of epinephrine, an $\alpha + \beta$–adrenergic agonist, or isoproterenol, a β-adrenergic agonist, was reported as a useful provocative test in LQTS more than 2 decades ago.[4] Before the discovery of the distinct genetic subtypes of LQTS, the responses to either epinephrine or isoproterenol were extremely heterogeneous and deemed impossible to interpret, and catecholamine stress testing once disappeared from the diagnostic workup of LQTS. However, the heterogeneous response is now understood to stem from the underlying genetic heterogeneity, and the gene-specific responses to epinephrine or isoproterenol can be exploited to expose different types of LQTS in its otherwise concealed state, particularly LQT1 syndrome. Because the heart rate is usually increased to more than 120 beats/min by isoproterenol infusion, especially by the use of bolus injection, it is often difficult to measure the QT interval precisely, due to an overlap of the next P wave on the terminal portion of T wave. Accordingly, epinephrine infusion has become a standard test, although isoproterenol is still used occasionally. In contrast to provocation studies using catecholamines, Viskin and colleagues[15] have shown that sudden heart rate oscillations precipitated by intravenous administration of adenosine may expose some patients with concealed LQTS, although genotype-specific responses have not been demonstrated. Compared with controls, patients with LQTS exhibited an exaggerated increase in the QT interval during adenosine-induced bradycardia.

The groups led by Ackerman[16] and Shimizu[17] pioneered a strategy of epinephrine provocative testing independently. Their 2 major protocols developed for epinephrine provocative testing include the escalating-dose protocol by Ackerman's group (Ackerman/Mayo Clinic protocol),[16] and the bolus injection followed by brief continuous infusion by Shimizu's group (Shimizu protocol).[17] Both protocols are extremely useful and safe, and overall are well tolerated, but should be viewed as diagnostic only, not prognostic. Induction of TdP or ventricular fibrillation is extremely uncommon in both protocols. Each protocol has some advantages and disadvantages with respect to the other. It is of importance that the diagnostic profiles gleaned from one protocol should not be applied to the other. It is critical to remember that the key determinant is epinephrine-mediated changes in the QT interval for the Ackerman protocol and epinephrine-mediated changes in the QTc interval for the Shimizu protocol.

Incremental, Escalating Epinephrine Infusion (Ackerman Protocol)

A 25-minute incremental, escalating infusion protocol (0.025–0.2 µg/kg/min) has been used by Ackerman and colleagues[16] in LQT1, LQT2, and LQT3 patients and in genotype-negative patients.[18,19] With epinephrine infusion at a low dose of 0.1 µg/kg/min or less, the median change of the QT interval was 78 milliseconds in LQT1, −4 milliseconds in LQT2, −58 milliseconds in LQT3, and −23 milliseconds in the genotype-negative patients. With this protocol, paradoxical QT prolongation, defined as a 30-millisecond increase in the QT (not QTc) interval during low-dose epinephrine infusion, was specific in the LQT1 patients (92%), but not in the LQT2 (13%), the LQT3 (0%), and the genotype-negative patients (18%). The paradoxical QT prolongation had a sensitivity of 92.5%, specificity of 86%, positive predictive value of 76%, and negative predictive value of 96% for LQT1 versus non-LQT1 status, and provides a presumptive, pregenetic clinical diagnosis of patients with LQT1 syndrome.

Better tolerance of the patient and a lower incidence of false-positive responses are major advantages of the escalating infusion protocol. On the other hand, this protocol seems less effective in exposing patients with LQT2 in comparison with the bolus protocol by Shimizu and colleagues described below. However, this disadvantage is reported to be partially overcome by focusing on the change of T-wave morphology during a low dose of epinephrine infusion. Khositseth and colleagues[19] reported that epinephrine-induced notched T wave was more indicative of LQT2 status.

Bolus Injection Followed by Brief Continuous Infusion (Shimizu Protocol)

The bolus protocol by Shimizu and colleagues was developed on the basis of a differential response of action potential duration (APD) and QT interval to sympathetic stimulation with isoproterenol between the experimental LQT1, LQT2, and LQT3 models using arterially perfused canine left ventricular wedge preparations.[20] In the LQT1 model, persistent prolongation of APD and QT interval at steady-state conditions of isoproterenol infusion was observed. Under normal conditions, β-adrenergic stimulation is expected to increase net outward repolarizing current, due to larger increase of outward currents, including Ca^{2+}-activated slow component of the delayed rectifier potassium current (I_{Ks}) and Ca^{2+}-activated chloride current ($I_{Cl(Ca)}$), than that of an inward current, Na^+/Ca^{2+} exchange current (I_{Na-Ca}), resulting in an abbreviation of APD and QT interval. A defect in I_{Ks}/Kv7.1 as seen in LQT1 could account for failure of β-adrenergic stimulation to abbreviate APD and QT interval, resulting in a persistent and paradoxical QT prolongation under sympathetic stimulation. In the LQT2 model, isoproterenol infusion was reported to initially prolong but then abbreviate APD and QT interval, probably because of an initial augmentation of I_{Na-Ca} and a subsequent stimulation of I_{Ks}. In the LQT3 model, on the other hand, isoproterenol infusion constantly abbreviated APD and QT interval as a result of a stimulation of I_{Ks}, because an inward late I_{Na} was augmented in this genotype. According to the differential responses of repolarization parameters to isoproterenol between the 3 models, the bolus protocol of epinephrine testing was expected not only to unmask concealed patients with LQTS but also to presumptively diagnose the 3 most common subtypes, namely LQT1, LQT2, and LQT3, by monitoring the temporal course of the QTc interval to epinephrine at peak effect following bolus injection and at steady-state effect during continuous infusion.

Clinical data using bolus protocol (Shimizu protocol; 0.1mg/kg bolus + 0.1/mg/kg/min infusion) suggested that sympathetic stimulation with epinephrine produces genotype-specific responses of the QTc (not QT) interval in patients with LQT1, LQT2, and LQT3 (**Fig. 1**).[21,22] Epinephrine remarkably prolonged the QTc interval at peak effect when the heart rate was maximally increased (1–2 minutes after the bolus injection), and the QTc remained prolonged during steady-state epinephrine effect (3–5 minutes) in patients with LQT1.[21,22] This steady-state effect with the Shimizu protocol likely corresponds with the paradoxical QT prolongation seen with the Ackerman protocol. The QTc interval was also prolonged at peak epinephrine effect (during bolus) in patients with LQT2, but returned to close to the baseline levels at steady-state epinephrine effect.[22] Compared with LQT1 and LQT2 patients, the QTc interval was less prolonged at peak epinephrine effect in the LQT3 patients, and was abbreviated below the baseline levels at steady-state

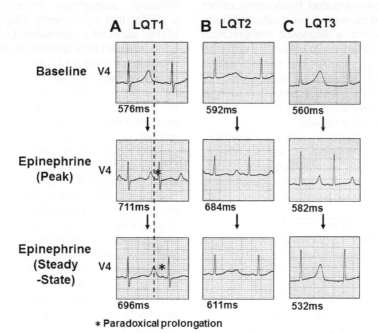

* Paradoxical prolongation

Fig. 1. Differential temporal change of the heart rate corrected QT (QTc) interval to epinephrine provocative testing in LQT1, LQT2, and LQT3 patients (Shimizu protocol). Shown are V4-lead ECG under baseline conditions, at peak and steady-state epinephrine effects in LQT1 (*A*), LQT2 (*B*), and LQT3 (*C*) patients using the Shimizu bolus and infusion protocol. The corrected QTc interval was prominently prolonged from 576 to 711 milliseconds at peak epinephrine effect, and remained prolonged at steady state (696 milliseconds) in the patient with LQT1. It is noteworthy that paradoxical QT prolongation was seen both at peak and steady-state epinephrine effects (*asterisk*). In the patient with LQT2, the QTc was also dramatically prolonged from 592 to 684 milliseconds at peak, but returned to the baseline level at steady state (611 milliseconds). It was much less prolonged (560–582 milliseconds) at peak in the LQT3 patient than in either the LQT1 or LQT2 patient, and returned to below the baseline level at steady state (532 milliseconds).

epinephrine effect.[22] The responses of the corrected T_{peak}-T_{end} interval reflecting transmural dispersion of repolarization (TDR) approximately paralleled those of the QT interval,[23] supporting the cellular basis for genotype-specific triggers for cardiac events.

Shimizu and colleagues[22] used the steady-state epinephrine effect, and reported improvement of clinical electrocardiographic diagnosis (sensitivity) from 68% to 87% in the 31 patients with LQT1 and from 83% to 91% in the 23 patients with LQT2, but not in the 6 patients with LQT3 (from 83% to 83%). The bolus protocol of epinephrine effectively predicts the underlying genotype of LQT1, LQT2, and LQT3 (**Fig. 2**).[22] The prolongation of QTc interval of 35 milliseconds or longer at steady-state epinephrine effect was able to differentiate LQT1 from LQT2, LQT3, or control patients with a predictive accuracy of 90% or greater. The prolongation of QTc interval of 80 milliseconds or longer at peak epinephrine effect was able to differentiate LQT2 from LQT3 or control patients with a predictive accuracy of 100%.

These gene-specific responses in both protocols are attenuated by β-blockers. If a patient displays epinephrine-induced bradycardia rather than the expected increase in heart rate, the study should be terminated, a diagnostic interpretation should not be rendered, and a period of monitored β-blocker washout should be considered. A caveat regarding epinephrine-accentuated U waves is in order also, as erroneous inclusion of such U waves during epinephrine infusion underlies some of the false positives.

Because molecular diagnosis is still unavailable for many patients throughout the world, unmasking concealed LQTS by the epinephrine provocative test can direct proper counseling and facilitate the use of β-blockers as well as the avoidance of QT-prolonging drugs. Furthermore, a presumptive, pregenetic diagnosis of LQT1, LQT2, or LQT3 based on the response to epinephrine can guide gene-specific treatment strategies. Clur and colleagues[24] recently evaluated the role of epinephrine testing (using the Shimizu protocol) in the diagnosis and management of children suspected of having congenital LQTS, who showed a borderline baseline QTc interval (441 ± 28 milliseconds) and nondiagnostic Schwartz score. The investigators reported that the epinephrine test cannot be used to diagnose genotype-positive LQTS, but suggested that it can be a tool to guide clinical decision making in a pediatric cohort with a suspicious LQTS phenotype. Because 25% of LQTS remains genetically elusive, the identification of patients with LQTS and an LQT1-like response to epinephrine, for example, may lead to the identification of novel LQTS-causing susceptibility genes.

EXERCISE STRESS TESTING

Although epinephrine provocative testing is a useful tool to correctly diagnose or unmask LQTS, especially concealed LQTS, it is usually conducted at LQTS specialty centers and typically requires a period of β-blocker washout. On the other hand, exercise stress testing, such as treadmill or bicycle testing with a variety of protocols, has long been more frequently used in both adult and pediatric cardiology centers.[25–27] Several studies reported the usefulness and genotype-specific responses of repolarization with exercise testing in LQTS patients, specifically in LQT1 and LQT2 genotypes.[28–30] Takenaka and colleagues[30] used treadmill exercise testing with a modified Bruce protocol and identified marked prolongation of QTc interval during exercise in LQT1 patients. By contrast, the identification of LQT2 patients was much more limited. However, they combined a qualitative assessment of T-wave morphology, that is, broad-based T waves in LQT1 patients and notched (bifid) T waves in LQT2 patients, and facilitated genotyping of the most common variants, LQT1 and LQT2 (**Fig. 3**). Wong and colleagues[31] also reported marked QTc-interval prolongation during exercise with treadmill and bicycle exercise testing in LQT1 patients, and only modest QTc-interval prolongation in LQT2 patients and genotype-negative control subjects. On the other hand, QT hysteresis, which was defined as the QT interval difference between exercise and 2 minutes into the recovery phase at similar heart rates, was more pronounced in

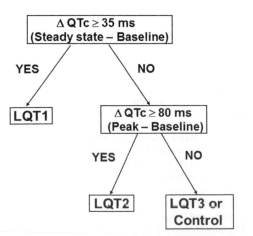

Fig. 2. Flow chart to predict genotype using bolus epinephrine provocative testing (Shimizu protocol).

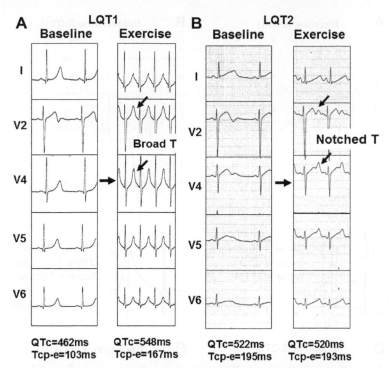

Fig. 3. Representative morphologic changes in the 5 leads of ECGs during treadmill exercise testing in LQT1 (*A*) and LQT2 (*B*) patients. During exercise, the LQT1 patient revealed a prominent prolongation in both corrected QT (QTc) interval (462–548 milliseconds) and T_{peak} to T_{end} (Tcp-e) interval (103–167 milliseconds) (*A*). The normal-appearing T patterns before exercise were changed to the broad-based pattern during exercise (*A*). On the contrary, a notch on the descending T-wave limb became prominent during exercise in LQT2 patient without significant prolongation of QTc and Tcp-e intervals (522–520 milliseconds and 195 to 193 milliseconds, respectively) (*B*). Measured values for QTc and Tcp-e are shown at the bottom of each column.

LQT2 patients than in LQT1 patients in their study.[31] Moreover, they also focused on the QTc changes with changes of posture (standing) before exercise as a simple, initial bedside screening test, and found that both LQT1 and LQT2 patients showed a greater prolongation of QTc interval with standing than control subjects. Wong and colleagues[31] speculated that the QTc prolongation with standing was attributable to a complex physiologic response involving sympathetic and parasympathetic mediated pathways that may lead to the recruitment of both I_{Ks} and I_{Kr} channels. Viskin and colleagues[32] also reported the usefulness of a bedside stand-up test for easily diagnosing LQTS. These investigators suggested that at maximal QT interval stretching, the time at which the end of the T wave gets nearest to the next P wave during transient sinus tachycardia after quick stand-up, the QTc-interval value identifies LQTS with 90% sensitivity and 86% specificity.

More recently, genotype-specific repolarization responses during recovery from exercise have received more focus. Chattha and colleagues[33] reported characteristic patterns of QT response after

exercise in LQT1 and LQT2 patients, which may have potential value both in diagnosing LQTS and in distinguishing LQT1 and LQT2 genotypes. LQT1 patients had the longest QTc interval during early recovery phase, after which the QTc interval decreased gradually during recovery, whereas LQT2 patients showed the lowest QTc interval at early recovery phase that increased thereafter into late recovery phase. Justin and colleagues[34] also evaluated the QTc interval during recovery phase in LQT1, LQT2, LQT3, and control subjects. These investigators suggested that either QTc interval of 460 milliseconds or longer during recovery phase or a paradoxical increase in QTc interval, defined as QTc recovery minus QTc baseline greater than or equal to 30 milliseconds (ΔQTc), distinguished LQT1 patients (manifest or concealed) from LQT2, LQT3, or control subjects.

TWENTY-FOUR-HOUR HOLTER RECORDING

Twenty-four-hour Holter recording is superior to the standard 12-lead ECG in detecting abnormal T-wave patterns by exploring a wide

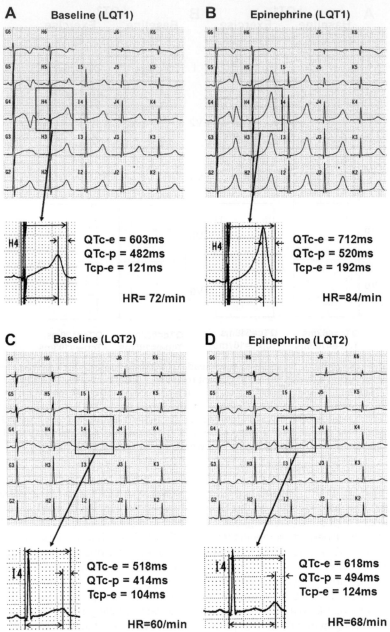

Fig. 4. Effects of epinephrine infusion on multiple-lead body surface potential ECGs in LQT1 (*A, B*) and LQT2 (*C, D*) patients. Shown are 24-lead ECGs (*G–K*: 2–6), which are selected from 87-lead body surface potential ECGs and are expected to reflect the potential from the left ventricular free wall under baseline conditions (*A, C*) and during epinephrine infusion (*B, D*). A representative ECG is shown on the lower trace in each panel (H4 in LQT1 and I4 in LQT2). In the LQT1 patient, the ECGs showed broad-based T waves commonly observed. Both the corrected QT$_{end}$ (QTc-e) and corrected QT$_{peak}$ (QTc-p) were prolonged (603 and 482 milliseconds, respectively), and the corrected T$_{peak}$ to T$_{end}$ (Tcp-e) was increased (121 milliseconds) under the baseline condition (*A*). Epinephrine produced a prominent prolongation in the QTc-e (712 milliseconds), but a mild prolongation in the QTc-p (520 milliseconds), resulting in a dramatic increase in the Tcp-e (192 milliseconds) (*B*). In the LQT2 patient, the ECGs showed low-amplitude T wave with a notched appearance commonly seen in LQT2 patients. The QTc-e and QTc-p were prolonged (518 and 414 milliseconds, respectively) and the Tcp-e was increased (104 milliseconds) under the baseline condition (*C*). Epinephrine produced a moderate prolongation in the QTc-e (618 milliseconds) and the QTc-p (494 milliseconds), resulting in a mild increase in the Tcp-e (124 milliseconds) (*D*).

range of cycle lengths over a period of 24 hours, although the numbers of ECG recordings are limited. Lupoglazoff and colleagues[35] monitored Holter recording in 133 LQT1 patients, 57 LQT2 patients, and 100 control subjects, and averaged T-wave templates were obtained at different cycle lengths. T-wave morphology was normal in most LQT1 and control subjects, whereas abnormal notched T waves were seen exclusively in LQT2 patients, with a prominent notches (a distinct protuberance above the apex) being most specific and often reflecting *KCNH2* core domain missense mutations. The Helsinki group focused more on the late repolarization phase of the T wave on 24-hour Holter recordings. Viitasalo and colleagues[36] reviewed 24-hour Holter recordings in 31 LQT1 patients, 28 LQT2 patients, and 31 unaffected family members, and measured the T-wave peak to T-wave end (TPE) interval, which is believed to reflect TDR and to serve as a substrate of TdP. These investigators reported that both median and maximal TPE intervals were greater in LQT2 than in LQT1 or unaffected patients, suggesting larger TDR in LQT2 than in LQT1 patients. More recently, Viitasalo and colleagues[37] measured maximal amplitude ratios between late (T2) and early (T1) T-wave peaks, based on both experimental and clinical evidence that the large T2 wave precedes the onset of TdP and that the ratio of T2 to T1 amplitude could be used as an ECG parameter to predict of TdP.[38–40] Maximal amplitude ratios between late and early T-wave peaks were higher in symptomatic than in asymptomatic patients in both LQT1 and LQT2 patients.[37] Multivariate analyses showed that the high T2 to T1 amplitude ratio was independently associated with symptoms, suggesting that this parameter carries a sign of the susceptibility for TdP in LQT1 and LQT2 patients.[37] Viitasalo and colleagues[41] also reported that β-blockers decreased the maximal T2 to T1 amplitude ratio as well as maximal TPE intervals in LQT1 patients, which may explain the favorable effects of β-blockers in LQT1. The analysis of T-wave morphology and repolarization parameters on 24-hour Holter recording has further advanced our understanding of the mechanism and the effects of drugs in patients with genotyped LQTS. However, diagnostic and prognostic values of this method are inferior to catecholamine provocative testing or exercise stress testing.

MULTIPLE-LEAD BODY SURFACE POTENTIAL MAPPING

Similar to 24-hour Holter recording, the analysis of repolarization parameters on multiple-lead body surface potential mapping has increased our knowledge on the mechanism and the effectiveness of drugs in LQTS patients. Whereas temporal changes of repolarization can be evaluated with Holter recording, recording of multiple-lead body surface potential ECGs enables the investigation of special heterogeneity of repolarization.[42,43] Tanabe and colleagues[44] recorded 87-lead body surface potential ECGs before and after epinephrine infusion in 13 LQT1, 6 LQT2, and 7 control patients. Epinephrine significantly increased the mean corrected QT_{end} (QTc-e) but not the mean corrected QT_{peak} (QTc-p), resulting in a significant increase in the mean corrected T_{peak} to T_{end} (Tcp-e), reflecting TDR in both LQT1 and LQT2 but not in control patients (**Fig. 4**). The epinephrine-induced increases in the mean QTc-e and Tcp-e were larger in LQT1 than in LQT2. Epinephrine also increased the maximum QTc-e but not the minimum QTc-e among 87 leads, producing a significant increase in the special dispersion of QTc-e in both LQT1 and LQT2 patients, but not in control patients. The increase in the special dispersion of QTc-e was larger in LQT1 than in LQT2 patients. These data suggested that sympathetic stimulation produces a greater increase in both TDR and spatial dispersion of repolarization (SDR) in LQT1 than in LQT2 syndrome, which may explain why LQT1 patients are more sensitive to sympathetic stimulation. Thereafter, Shimizu and colleagues[23] used 87-lead body surface potential ECGs, and compared the effects of a β-blocker on TDR and SDR between LQT1 and LQT2 patients. Propranolol in the absence of epinephrine significantly prolonged the mean QTc-p but not the mean QTc-e, thus decreasing the mean Tcp-e (TDR) in LQT1 patients more than that in LQT2 patients. Propranolol completely suppressed the influence of epinephrine in prolonging the mean QTc-e, maximum QTc-e, and minimum QTc-e, as well as increasing the mean Tcp-e and special dispersion of QTc-e in both groups. The investigators concluded that β-blockade under normal sympathetic tone produces a greater decrease in TDR in LQT1 than in LQT2 patients, explaining the superior effectiveness of β-blockers in LQT1 over LQT2. β-Blockers also suppress the influence of sympathetic stimulation in increasing TDR and SDR equally in LQT1 and LQT2 syndrome.

REFERENCES

1. Schwartz PJ, Periti M, Malliani A. The long QT syndrome. Am Heart J 1975;89:378–90.
2. Schwartz PJ, Moss AJ, Vincent GM, et al. Diagnostic criteria for the long QT syndrome: an update. Circulation 1993;88:782–4.

3. Moss AJ, Schwartz PJ, Crampton RS, et al. The long QT syndrome: a prospective international study. Circulation 1985;71:17–21.

4. Schechter E, Freeman CC, Lazzara R. Afterdepolarizations as a mechanism for the long QT syndrome: electrophysiologic studies of a case. J Am Coll Cardiol 1984;3:1556–61.

5. Priori SG. The fifteen years of discoveries that shaped molecular electrophysiology: time for appraisal. Circ Res 2010;107:451–6.

6. Ackerman MJ, Mohler PJ. Defining a new paradigm for human arrhythmia syndromes: phenotypic manifestations of gene mutations in ion channel- and transporter-associated proteins. Circ Res 2010; 107:457–65.

7. Napolitano C, Antzelevitch C. Phenotypical manifestations of mutations in the genes encoding subunits of the cardiac voltage-dependent L-type calcium channel. Circ Res 2011;108:607–18.

8. Wilde AA, Brugada R. Phenotypical manifestations of mutations in the genes encoding subunits of the cardiac sodium channel. Circ Res 2011;108: 884–97.

9. Shimizu W, Horie M. Phenotypic manifestations of mutations in genes encoding subunits of cardiac potassium channels. Circ Res 2011;109:97–109.

10. Priori SG, Napolitano C, Schwartz PJ, et al. Association of long QT syndrome loci and cardiac events among patients treated with beta-blockers. JAMA 2004;292:1341–4.

11. Vincent GM, Timothy KW, Leppert M, et al. The spectrum of symptoms and QT intervals in carriers of the gene for the long-QT syndrome. N Engl J Med 1992;327:846–52.

12. Priori SG, Napolitano C, Schwartz PJ. Low penetrance in the Long-QT syndrome. Clinical impact. Circulation 1999;99:529–33.

13. Swan H, Saarinen K, Kontula K, et al. Evaluation of QT interval duration and dispersion and proposed clinical criteria in diagnosis of long QT syndrome in patients with a genetically uniform type of LQT1. J Am Coll Cardiol 1998;32:486–91.

14. Priori SG, Schwartz PJ, Napolitano C, et al. Risk stratification in the long-QT syndrome. N Engl J Med 2003;348:1866–74.

15. Viskin S, Rosso R, Rogowski O, et al. Provocation of sudden heart rate oscillation with adenosine exposes abnormal QT responses in patients with long QT syndrome: a bedside test for diagnosing long QT syndrome. Eur Heart J 2006;27:469–75.

16. Ackerman MJ, Khositseth A, Tester DJ, et al. Epinephrine-induced QT interval prolongation: a gene-specific paradoxical response in congenital long QT syndrome. Mayo Clin Proc 2002;77:413–21.

17. Noda T, Takaki H, Kurita T, et al. Gene-specific response of dynamic ventricular repolarization to sympathetic stimulation in LQT1, LQT2 and LQT3

forms of congenital long QT syndrome. Eur Heart J 2002;23:975–83.

18. Vyas H, Hejlik J, Ackerman MJ. Epinephrine QT stress testing in the evaluation of congenital long-QT syndrome: diagnostic accuracy of the paradoxical QT response. Circulation 2006;113:1385–92.

19. Khositseth A, Hejlik J, Shen WK, et al. Epinephrine-induced T-wave notching in congenital long QT syndrome. Heart Rhythm 2005;2:141–6.

20. Shimizu W, Antzelevitch C. Differential response to beta-adrenergic agonists and antagonists in LQT1, LQT2 and LQT3 models of the long QT syndrome. J Am Coll Cardiol 2000;35:778–86.

21. Shimizu W, Noda T, Takaki H, et al. Epinephrine unmasks latent mutation carriers with LQT1 form of congenital long QT syndrome. J Am Coll Cardiol 2003;41:633–42.

22. Shimizu W, Noda T, Takaki H, et al. Diagnostic value of epinephrine test for genotyping LQT1, LQT2 and LQT3 forms of congenital long QT syndrome. Heart Rhythm 2004;1:276–83.

23. Shimizu W, Tanabe Y, Aiba T, et al. Differential effects of β-blockade on dispersion of repolarization in absence and presence of sympathetic stimulation between LQT1 and LQT2 forms of congenital long QT syndrome. J Am Coll Cardiol 2002;39:1984–91.

24. Clur SA, Chockalingam P, Filippini LH, et al. The role of the epinephrine test in the diagnosis and management of children suspected of having congenital long QT syndrome. Pediatr Cardiol 2010;31: 462–8.

25. Shimizu W, Ohe T, Kurita T, et al. Differential response of QTU interval to exercise, isoproterenol, and atrial pacing in patients with congenital long QT syndrome. Pacing Clin Electrophysiol 1991;14: 1966–70.

26. Kawade M, Ohe T, Arakaki Y, et al. Abnormal response to exercise, face immersion and isoproterenol in children with the long QT syndrome. Pacing Clin Electrophysiol 1995;18:2128–34.

27. Swan H, Saarinen K, Kontula K, et al. Rate adaptation of QT intervals during and after exercise in children with congenital long QT syndrome. Eur Heart J 1998;19:508–13.

28. Swan H, Viitasalo M, Piippo K, et al. Sinus node function and ventricular repolarization during exercise stress test in long QT syndrome patients with KvLQT1 and HERG potassium channel defects. J Am Coll Cardiol 1999;34:823–9.

29. Paavonen KJ, Swan H, Piippo K, et al. Response of the QT interval to mental and physical stress in types LQT1 and LQT2 of the long QT syndrome. Heart 2001;86:39–44.

30. Takonaka K, Ai T, Shimizu W, et al. Exercise stress test amplifies genotype-phenotype correlation in the LQT1 and LQT2 forms of the long QT syndrome. Circulation 2003;107:838–44.

31. Wong JA, Gula LJ, Klein GJ, et al. Utility of treadmill testing in identification and genotype prediction in long-QT syndrome. Circ Arrhythm Electrophysiol 2010;3:120–5.

32. Viskin S, Postema PG, Bhuiyan ZA, et al. The response of the QT interval to the brief tachycardia provoked by standing: a bedside test for diagnosing long QT syndrome. J Am Coll Cardiol 2010; 55:1955–61.

33. Chattha IS, Sy RW, Yee R, et al. Utility of the recovery electrocardiogram after exercise: a novel indicator for the diagnosis and genotyping of long QT syndrome? Heart Rhythm 2010;7:906–11.

34. Horner JM, Horner MM, Ackerman MJ. The diagnostic utility of recovery phase QTc during treadmill exercise stress testing in the evaluation of long QT syndrome. Heart Rhythm 2011;8(11):1698–704.

35. Lupoglazoff JM, Denjoy I, Berthet M, et al. Notched T waves on Holter recordings enhance detection of patients with LQt2 (HERG) mutations. Circulation 2001;103:1095–101.

36. Viitasalo M, Oikarinen L, Swan H, et al. Ambulatory electrocardiographic evidence of transmural dispersion of repolarization in patients with long-QT syndrome type 1 and 2. Circulation 2002;106: 2473–8.

37. Viitasalo M, Oikarinen L, Swan H, et al. Ratio of late to early T-wave peak amplitude in 24-h electrocardiographic recordings as indicator of symptom history in patients with long-QT syndrome types 1 and 2. J Am Coll Cardiol 2006;47:112–20.

38. Gbadebo TD, Trimble RW, Khoo MS, et al. Calmodulin inhibitor W-7 unmasks a novel electrocardiographic parameter that predicts initiation of torsade de pointes. Circulation 2002;105:770–4.

39. Mazur A, Roden DM, Anderson ME. Systemic administration of calmodulin antagonist W-7 or protein kinase A inhibitor H-8 prevents torsade de pointes in rabbits. Circulation 1999;100:2437–42.

40. Shimizu W, Ohe T, Kurita T, et al. Early afterdepolarizations induced by isoproterenol in patients with congenital long QT syndrome. Circulation 1991;84: 1915–23.

41. Viitasalo M, Oikarinen L, Swan H, et al. Effects of beta-blocker therapy on ventricular repolarization documented by 24-h electrocardiography in patients with type 1 long-QT syndrome. J Am Coll Cardiol 2006;48:747–53.

42. Shimizu W, Kamakura S, Kurita T, et al. Influence of epinephrine, propranolol and atrial pacing on spatial distribution of recovery time measured by body surface mapping in congenital long QT syndrome. J Cardiovasc Electrophysiol 1997;8:1102–14.

43. Shimizu W, Kamakura S, Ohe T, et al. Diagnostic value of recovery time measured by body surface mapping in patients with congenital long QT syndrome. Am J Cardiol 1994;74:780–5.

44. Tanabe Y, Inagaki M, Kurita T, et al. Sympathetic stimulation produces a greater increase in both transmural and spatial dispersion of repolarization in LQT1 than LQT2 forms of congenital long QT syndrome. J Am Coll Cardiol 2001;37:911–9.

Age and Gender Modulation of the Long QT Syndrome Phenotype

Ohad Ziv, MD, Elizabeth S. Kaufman, MD*

KEYWORDS

- Long QT • Gender • Repolarization • Sudden death
- Syncope • Hormonal

Recent literature points to a complex relationship between gender, age, and long QT syndrome (LQTS), both congenital and acquired. Understanding of this complex relationship is essential for the clinician because it plays an important role in clinical outcomes. Importantly, both syncope and sudden death in LQTS are affected by the presence or absence of sex hormones. In this article, we begin with a review of the manner in which age and gender affect electrocardiographic (ECG) measurements of repolarization and therefore the QT interval. We detail the effects of age and gender on clinical outcomes and review how these modulations drive treatment recommendations. We also discuss basic research that has recently begun to shed light on these clinical phenomena and may give insight into potential future treatments.

REVIEW OF HUMAN SEX HORMONE PHYSIOLOGY

To understand how gender and age modulate the QT interval and therefore LQTS, we first briefly summarize the progression of human sex hormone exposure in men and women throughout the basic stages of life. In men, the testes secrete androgens, including androstenedione; dihydrotestosterone; and, much more abundantly, testosterone. Estrogens are produced in men as well, although at an estimated 20% of that in a nonpregnant woman. The majority of the estrogen in men comes from conversion of testosterone and androstenediol to estrogens in somatic tissue.[1,2]

The interstitial cells of Leydig within the testes begin to produce testosterone at around the seventh week of embryonic life. Ten weeks after birth, testosterone secretion shuts down and little measurable testosterone is produced until puberty. At puberty, there is a steep increase to a peak production of nearly 7000 μg/d of testosterone in young adulthood. Thereafter, there is a steady decline of production reaching 20% to 50% of peak values by age 80 years.[1,3,4]

In women, the theca cells of the ovary produce androstenedione and testosterone, although the majority of the androgens produced undergo conversion within the ovary into, primarily, estrogens. Thus, ovaries produce only 7% of the androgens seen in males. The granulosa cells produce estrogens and progestins. Estrogen production is at a minimum in women until the monthly hormonal cycles begin at puberty. During young adulthood, estrogen secretion cycles between 100 and 300 μg/d.[1] At menopause, there is a steady decline of estrogen in a fluctuating pattern until a minimum is reached. Decline in progesterone production is more rapid.[5–8] Furthermore, androgen levels decrease dramatically, with onset of reduction occurring before menopause. The androgens that are produced are heavily converted

Conflict of interest: The authors have nothing to disclose.
Heart and Vascular Research Center, MetroHealth Campus of Case Western Reserve University, Hamann 3rd Floor, 2500 MetroHealth Drive, Cleveland, OH 44109-1998, USA
* Corresponding author.
E-mail address: ekaufman@metrohealth.org

Card Electrophysiol Clin 4 (2012) 39–51
doi:10.1016/j.ccep.2011.12.003

to estrogens in adipose tissue. Thus, the postmeno-pausal hormonal state is one of low progesterone and androgen levels and reduced but measurable estrogen levels.

During pregnancy, estrogen and progesterone levels increase significantly as a result of placental secretion. Estrogen increases to a level of 30 times more than normal levels, although the potency of the primary estrogen produced (estriol) is significantly lower than that of estradiol. Progesterone is also produced in vast quantities during pregnancy, averaging 0.25 gm/d toward the end of pregnancy. In the postpartum period, there is a rapid decline of hormones to levels lower than the nonpregnant state. Breastfeeding prolongs this suppressed state.[1,9,10]

AGE AND GENDER EFFECTS ON CLINICAL ECG

In the 1920s, Bazett noted that the QT interval was longer in women. Early population studies of repolarization in humans as measured by the QT interval revealed longer QT intervals in women than in men. With ECG data from more than 400 normal men and women with a mean age of 40 years, Merri and colleagues[11] demonstrated that the mean QTc interval was 12 milliseconds (ms) longer in woman than men. Evidence of sex hormone effect on QTc is observed when QTc is compared at the various phases of the ovulatory cycle in women after autonomic blockade with atropine and propranolol. During the follicular phase, marked by an increase in estrogen alone, women have a longer QTc interval than in the luteal phase, which is associated with an increase in progesterone levels and a more modest increase in estrogen levels.[12] This finding was echoed by Rodriguez and colleagues[13] who showed that the QT response to ibutilide infusion varied depending on subjects' menstrual cycle. Again, the luteal phase was protective against QT prolongation in these female subjects. More recent population data underscore the underlying hormonal effect on QT. Kadish and colleagues[14] demonstrated that QT intervals of postmenopausal women treated with estrogen-only hormone replacement therapy were significantly longer than those of women treated with estrogen-progesterone combined therapy.

Age adds an additional dimension to the gender-QT interaction. During infancy and childhood, the QTc interval appears no different between boys and girls. With the onset of puberty, the QTc shortens in men by 20 ms (**Fig. 1**), whereas in women it appears stable through sexual maturation.[15] The longer QTc in women appears to be maintained throughout adulthood,[16,17] although the difference diminishes significantly after age 50 years.[17] Importantly, both

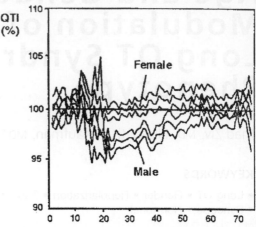

Fig. 1. Effect of age on QT in men and women. QT index (QTi = QT measured/QT expected) plotted for men and women from birth to age 70 years. For both genders, the 3 lines plotted represent the mean QTi (*middle line*) along with the upper and lower standard deviations of the mean. Of note, at puberty, the QT index of men is significantly reduced compared with that of women. The QT index of men and women do not overlap again until after age 50 years. (*From* Rautaharju PM, Zhou SH, Wong S, et al. Sex differences in the evolution of the electrocardiographic QT interval with age. Can J Cardiol 1992;8(7): 693; with permission.)

men and women see prolongation of their QT interval with increase in age in late adulthood. The mean QTc appears to increase 1 ms for each decade of life after age 50 years.[18]

Several other important differences are seen with respect to repolarization and gender. First, the shape of the T wave changes with respect to gender and exposure to sex hormones. Women have lower-amplitude T waves by 25% compared with that in men.[19] Furthermore, both the ascending and descending limbs of the T-wave slope are flatter in women than in men. This pattern appears to reverse when comparing women with virilization syndrome with castrated men.[20,21] On 24-hour Holter monitoring, the QT-RR relationship is different between men and women. Regardless of which aspect of the T-wave is used, the slope of the QT-RR linear regression is steeper in women.[22] Recent data confirm this finding (**Fig. 2**).[23] These differences reflect important physiologic differences between cardiac repolarization in men and women. In the next section, we explore the basic mechanisms underlying these differences that directly affect the phenotype in LQTS.

BASIC MECHANISMS

Receptors to estrogen, androgens, and progesterone have all been demonstrated in cardiac

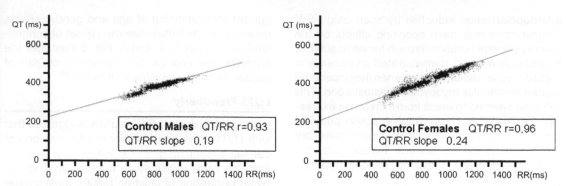

Fig. 2. QT-RR relationship in healthy young adults. QT intervals (in milliseconds) plotted against the R-R interval from healthy young adults without intervention. Panel on left shows the relationship in men and panel on right shows the relationship in women. Of note, the slope of the QT-RR relationship in women is significantly steeper than in men. (*Adapted from* Genovesi S, Zaccaria D, Rossi E, et al. Effects of exercise training on heart rate and QT interval in healthy young individuals: are there gender differences? Europace 2007;9(1):58; with permission.)

ventricular myocytes in several animal models.[17,24–27] These receptors result in actions on ventricular repolarization on both a transcriptional and nontranscriptional manner (**Table 1**).

In animal models, at longer R-R intervals, estrogen prolongs action potential duration in ventricular myocytes.[17] In acute studies, estrogen blocks I_{Kr} in guinea pig ventricular myocytes.[28] An effect of estrogen on transcription of RNA message for HERG has not been demonstrated.[17] Thus the effect of estrogen prolonging the action potential duration, and therefore the QT interval, seems to be at a nongenomic level. Therefore, when stimulating ventricular myocytes at long intervals, when repolarization is more dependent on I_{Kr}, it is observed that estrogen produces significant action potential duration prolongation in rabbit myocytes. However, as stimulation intervals shorten and I_{Ks} contribution to repolarization increases, the blockade of I_{Kr} has less effect on action potential duration because of the increase of repolarization reserve. When taking these effects into account, we can explain the steeper slope of the QT-RR relationship in women as an estrogen effect. This effect is seen in animal models[17,29,30] as well as in women as described earlier. Paradoxically, at higher

doses, estrogen increases I_{Ks} current, resulting in an opposing effect on the QT at these levels.[31] Therefore, a differential effect of estrogen on the QT interval in a dose-response manner may be expected. Higher levels of circulating estrogen, such as during pregnancy, may in fact have less prolonging effects on QT interval than the lower estrogen levels during ovulatory cycles. These differences and the potential clinical effects are discussed in detail later.

Progesterone, in contrast, shortens the action potential duration of cardiac myocytes. Nakamura and colleagues[25] demonstrated upregulation of I_{Ks} current acutely in guinea pig ventricular myocytes exposed to progesterone. The mechanism of this action seems to be through a nitric oxide signal transduction-dependent pathway. The same group demonstrated that although at basal conditions progesterone had no measurable effect on I_{CaL}, under a condition of increased cyclic adenosine monophosphate levels, such as a high adrenergic state, progesterone significantly reduced I_{CaL} current. Both of these actions shortened the action potential duration and reduced the likelihood of early afterdepolarization in the modeling of ventricular myocytes with long action potential duration.[25]

Testosterone also acts on the action potential of ventricular myocytes. In male rabbits after orchiectomy, the prolongation seen with exposure to dofetilide is reduced when the animals are pretreated with testosterone.[17] Like estrogen and progesterone, testosterone seems to have a nongenomic effect, in this case, induction of I_{Kr} increase.[32] Thus, multiple studies have demonstrated that testosterone acts to reduce the action potential duration prolongation seen with exposure to I_{Kr} blockers and to reduce the likelihood of early

Table 1
Summary of data of sex hormone effects on ventricular repolarization

Hormone	I_{Kr}	I_{Ks}	I_{CaL}	QT interval
Estrogen	↑	↑ (at high dose only)	↑ (?)	↑
Progesterone	↔	↑	↓	↓
Testosterone	↓	↔	↑ (?)	↓

afterdepolarization induction by such drugs.[33,34] Testosterone may have opposing effects on the action potential duration through genomic actions. Er and colleagues[35] demonstrated an increase in inward L-type calcium current when they incubated human ventricular myocytes in testosterone. This increase seemed to result from increase in expression of Ca(v) 1.2. Thus, although action potential duration shortening effects of testosterone are direct effects on I_{Kr} current, testosterone has genomic effects on I_{CaL} that may prolong the action potential duration.

With the development of transgenic rabbits with LQTS type 1 and type 2 (LQT1 and LQT2), one group has embarked on deciphering the effects of each of these gonadotropic hormones specifically on female rabbits with either LQT1 or LQT2. In their initial article describing the LQT2 model, Brunner and colleagues[30] report a nearly 50% mortality due to polymorphic ventricular tachycardia. The deaths seemed to cluster in the postpartum period. This model mimics some of the key features of hormone effects in women with LQTS (as we describe in the next section) and may play a significant role in further understanding these complex interactions.

CLINICAL MANIFESTATIONS OF AGE AND GENDER EFFECTS IN CONGENITAL LQTS

There are clear gender differences in risk of cardiac events: syncope, aborted cardiac arrest, or sudden death.[36] In this section, we review the current understanding of age and gender effects on events in the 3 most common types of congenital LQTS: types 1, 2, and 3. **Fig. 3** illustrates the complex age and gender interaction on risk of cardiac events in patients with LQTS.[37]

LQTS Prepuberty

Initial data from the LQTS registry suggested that with LQT1, boys had a higher risk for syncope or cardiac arrest than girls.[38] In a subsequent report from the same registry with a much larger genotyped population of children (>800), male gender was an independent risk factor for syncope or cardiac arrest regardless of the genotype.[39]

From this important finding arises the question of what there is about the male gender that increases the risk for events. Goldenberg and colleagues[39] suggest that the difference may be multifactorial, including "environmental, genetic and hormonal effects." If the increased risk arose from disproportionate involvement in activity level or involvement in athletic competition, one would expect that data from several decades ago might show a more robust difference between boys and girls than more recent data because in recent years, girls frequently participate in competitive athletic sports. The role played by hormonal effects during childhood on this gender difference in LQT-related events remains unclear. It is possible that testosterone withdrawal in early childhood in boys is associated with increased risk of long QT-related events.

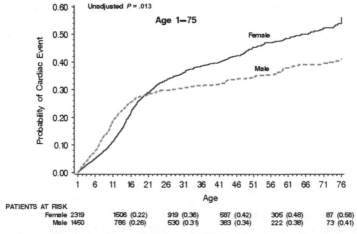

Fig. 3. Probability of a first cardiac event from age 1 through 75 years by gender. The dashed line shows the probability of a first cardiac event in men. This curve rises steeply during childhood but becomes flatter in late adolescence/early adulthood. The solid line shows the probability of a first cardiac event in women. During childhood, the risk in girls is lower than the risk in boys. However, in late adolescence/early adulthood the lines cross, and the risk remains higher in women than in men throughout adulthood. The curve representing risk in women remains steeper than the curve representing risk in men, with further separation of the curves throughout life. (*From* Goldenberg I, Moss AJ, Zareba W. Time-dependent gender differences in the clinical course of patients with the congenital long-QT syndrome. In: Wang P, Hsia H, Al-Ahmad A, et al, editors. Ventricular arrhythmias and sudden cardiac death mechanism. Malden (MA): Blackwell Publishing Inc.; 2008. p. 30, with permission.)

LQTS Postpuberty

Postpuberty, the gender effect reverses with a significantly increased risk of cardiac events in women compared with men. Sauer and colleagues[40] demonstrated that between the ages of 18 and 40 years, female gender was an independent predictor of LQTS-related events. It was also an independent risk factor for aborted cardiac arrest or sudden death. By age 40 years, women with congenital LQTS had a 40% rate of a cardiac event compared with 10% in men. The curves representing cumulative probability of life-threatening LQTS events for men and women separate early postpuberty, and although the men's event rate seems to level off, the women's cumulative event rate continues to increase, suggesting a persistent role for gender in altering risk for events throughout this period (**Fig. 4**).

The emergence of increased risk after puberty in women can be explained by hormonal effects on the QT, action potential duration, and delayed repolarization currents. First, the QTc of men decreases after puberty because of the induction of I_{Kr} by testosterone. Thus, men with LQTS may be protected from development of torsades de pointes. Second, estrogen exposure at postpuberty levels for women reduces I_{Kr} and therefore prolongs action potential duration, increasing the likelihood of an LQTS-related event.

The fact that female gender is a predictor of events independent of QT interval suggests that more is at play in this phenomenon than mere prolongation of the QT interval in women compared with men. Wasserstrom and colleagues[41] describe a significant difference in calcium transients of female rat compared with male rat intact hearts. Calcium transients in female rats were of lower amplitude and longer duration those in male rats. The investigators also describe a greater heterogeneity in single cell measurement of calcium transients. Thus, alteration in calcium cycling as a result of differential sex hormone exposure may contribute to the increased risk in women with long QT. Odening and colleagues[42] have demonstrated that in a rabbit model of LQT2, exposure to estrogen reverses the usual base to apex gradient of long to short action potential duration. This finding suggests the potential role of sex hormones in modulating heterogeneity in action potential duration and thus the substrate required for lethal LQTS-related arrhythmias.

GENOTYPE-SPECIFIC EFFECT OF PUBERTY IN CONGENITAL LONG QT

Given these changes introduced by sex hormones, it would be predicted that the increased event risk in women would be independent of LQTS genotype. However, although Zareba and colleagues[43] demonstrated an increase greater than 3-fold in risk for LQTS-related events in women with LQT1 and LQT2 in the 18- to 40-year-old patient population, they did not see a similar result in the patients with LQTS type 3 (LQT3). Preliminary data from the LQTS registry show no difference in LQT3 male and female events after puberty (Kaufman and colleagues, unpublished data). This distinctive behavior of LQT3 is an interesting phenomenon that may stem from differences in mechanism of

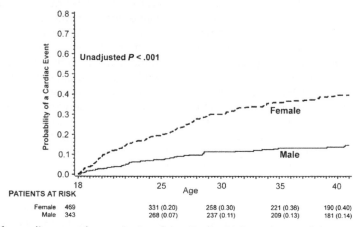

Fig. 4. Probability of a cardiac event by gender in adults. Kaplan-Meier estimate of the cumulative probability of aborted cardiac arrest (ACA) or LQTS-related sudden death after age 18 years among patients with mutation-confirmed LQTS according to gender. The *P* value was computed with the log-rank test, unadjusted for covariates. The numbers of subjects remaining at risk are given at 5-year intervals beginning at age 25 years, with the numbers in parentheses indicating the cumulative probability of a cardiac event at the specified age. (*From* Sauer AJ, Moss AJ, McNitt S, et al. Long QT syndrome in adults. J Am Coll Cardiol 2007;49(3):335; with permission.)

arrhythmia formation among the genotypes and needs to be further investigated.

The interaction of gender and genotype is likely more complex for all genotypes than previously thought. Recently published data[44] comparing pore with nonpore mutations in men and women with LQT2 showed that women were at higher risk of an LQTS-related event than men, but the risk of an event in women was not related to the location of the mutation. Men, on the other hand, had a 2-fold higher risk of an event if they possessed a pore mutation compared with a nonpore mutation. Pore mutations usually result in a greater reduction in I_{Kr} than nonpore mutations.[45–47] Nonpore mutations reduce I_{Kr} but may require a second "hit"[48] in repolarization reserve to manifest clinically.[38]

In this context, it is possible that the reduction in I_{Kr} by estrogen along with lack of induction of I_{Kr} by testosterone renders female gender the second "hit" in repolarization reserve. Thus, nonpore mutations are sufficient to cause cardiac events when they occur in women. In men, who lack this second hit, a nonpore mutation may not be sufficient on its own, and a lower risk for cardiac events is seen. We are likely just beginning to understand the intricacies of gender, sex hormones, and genotype variations on the risk for cardiac events. More data and modeling are required to fully unmask this interaction.

CLINICAL EFFECTS OF HORMONE FLUCTUATIONS
Pregnancy and the Postpartum Period

If hormones underlie the gender-specific changes in risk for cardiac events in LQTS, then it can be expected that the changes in the hormone exposure that occur within the lifetime of a woman would also have an effect on her risk for an event during specific periods. During pregnancy and the postpartum period, women are subject to some of the largest changes in hormonal exposure in their lifetime. Therefore, it is not surprising that vast changes in risk for cardiac events exist within this period. Seth and colleagues[49] reported that in the 391 women in the LQTS registry who gave birth between 1980 and 2003, the 9-month postpartum period presented a 2.7-fold increase in risk for any cardiac event and a 4-fold increase for life-threatening arrhythmic events. In inspecting the graph of cumulative risk of events for this population of women from the time of conception of their child to 48 months after conception (**Fig. 5**), a steep increase can be appreciated in event rate that occurs after birth of the child that persists up to a year after the birth. This finding was most robust

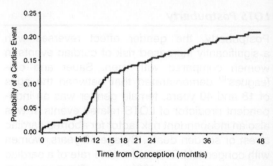

Fig. 5. Probability of a cardiac event by time from conception. Cumulative probability of a first cardiac event during 48 months after first conception after age 15 years in 391 women with LQTS who had a live birth between 1980 and 2003. (*From* Seth R, Moss AJ, McNitt S, et al. Long QT syndrome and pregnancy. J Am Coll Cardiol 2007;49(10):1095; with permission.)

in women with LQT2 and confirms similar findings in this genotype by others.[50] The increase in risk in the postpartum period was present, but less pronounced, in women with LQT1. In women with LQT3, pregnancy itself seemed to be the time of highest risk. However, the investigators caution against basing any conclusions on these data because the study only included 12 genotyped women with LQT3.

When comparing the prepregnant state, defined as the period from age 15 years to the first pregnancy, to the pregnant state, this cohort of women had a lower rate of all cardiac events during pregnancy.[49] Life-threatening events, however, were no different in the prepregnancy and pregnant states. The high levels of estrogen during pregnancy may be sufficiently high to induce I_{Ks}. This potential change, together with an increase in I_{Ks} from the high levels of progesterone, likely increases repolarization reserve in the pregnant state and may protect against cardiac events during this period. With the withdrawal of estrogen and progesterone in the postpartum state, the period of increased repolarization reserve ends and an increase in event rates is seen. This explanation, however, falls short of explaining why postpartum rates of events far exceed prepuberty event rates in women. The slowing of heart rate postpartum may be a major contributor to the increase in events postpartum. Support for this lies in the fact that in women with LQT2, where mechanism of arrhythmia is pause dependent,[51] we see by far the largest increase in risk of postpartum events.[49] In addition, multiple other physiologic changes occur postpartum, including exposure to prolactin and oxytocin. Effects of these hormones on LQTS and the QT interval have not been investigated. Social stressors and increase in sympathetic stimulation postpartum may play a role in the increase in events.

Menstrual Cycle

As described earlier, changes in hormone exposure during the phases of the menstrual cycle do affect the QT interval. They also have been shown to affect the rates of drug-induced torsades de pointes (discussed in a later section). In congenital LQTS, at present, there are no data linking events to a specific time during the menstrual cycle. Presumably, the QT on ECG and the risk of long QT–related events would be higher in women with long QT during the follicular phase with exposure to estrogen alone. During the luteal phase, when women are exposed to progesterone as well, a reduction in events would be expected. Although data supporting this do not currently exist, monthly variations in the QT interval in women with LQTS may have diagnostic and prognostic ramifications. We discuss these in detail in the "Diagnostic and Treatment Considerations" section later.

Menopause

With the onset of menopause, again women experience large shifts in hormone exposure. As one would expect, these shifts result in significant changes in the phenotype manifested by women with LQTS. Recently, Buber and colleagues[52] published data on postmenopausal women from the LQTS registry. This prospective study followed more than 150 women with LQT1 and more than 130 women with LQT2 through their transition to the postmenopausal state. In women with LQT2, menopause was associated with an 8-fold increase in the risk of syncope compared with the reproductive years. In contrast, LQT1 women had a nonsignificant reduction in syncopal events after menopause compared with their reproductive years. Estrogen replacement therapy in either genotype did not seem to change the rate of events.

The investigators suggest several possible explanations for these findings. First, they point to the hormonal changes associated with menopause, including the loss of testosterone and the maintenance of low levels of estrogen from extragonadal sources. Both of these changes result in reduction in I_{Kr}, rather than any effect on I_{Ks}. The investigators speculate that the lack of change of I_{Ks} may explain the effect on LQT2 rather than LQT1. They also remind us that the sustained high adrenergic state required for arrhythmias in LQT1 is perhaps achieved less frequently in this older population, whereas the bradycardia associated

with LQT2 arrhythmias is more prevalent in this age group.

This latter explanation suggests that age itself may play a significant role in the differential effects seen in women with postmenopausal LQT1 and LQT2. In fact, this difference seems to hold up when investigating the risk of events after age 40 years among various genotypes.[53] In a study including men and women with LQT1, LQT2, and LQT3, compared with genotype-negative family members, patients with LQT3 had a nearly 5-fold increased risk of cardiac events, and patients with LQT2 had a 2.5-fold increase in events. In contrast, patients with LQT1 had an event rate similar to the genotype-negative control group. This result, which echoes the findings in postmenopausal women with LQT1 and LQT2, suggests that age-related changes in heart rate and perhaps behavior may play a significant role in reduction of events in patients with LQT1 in later adulthood.

Congenital Long QT and Increasing Age: Effects of Acquired Disease

It appears that after age 40 years, female gender is no longer an independent risk factor for LQTS-related events. Goldenberg and colleagues[53] further investigated this phenomenon through a subgroup analysis comparing the hazard ratio of events in women compared with men in age groups 41 to 60 years and 61 to 75 years and stratified by QTc. Gender did not seem to affect risk, with the exception of a higher risk in men in the 61 to 75 age group with QTc less than 440 ms (**Fig. 6**). The investigators suggest that the increased risk of LQTS events because of female gender was matched by the greater risk of coronary disease and acquired cardiac disease in men in this age group. Still, when comparing all patients with positive LQTS genotype with family members with negative genotype in this same age group with presumably the same exposure to acquired cardiac disease, a positive genotype still carried a significantly greater risk of a major cardiac event. Genotype-positive patients demonstrated a cumulative risk of 20% for aborted cardiac arrest or sudden death by age 75 years. This was twice the rate of their genotype-negative family members. Thus, although gender becomes less significant after age 40 years, long QT genotype still increases risk.

One of the diseases more prevalent in patients older than 40 years is diabetes. Although diabetes increases mortality, this is independent of any effect on LQTS-related events.[54] In fact, QTc does not seem to be different among patients with congenital LQTS with or without diabetes.

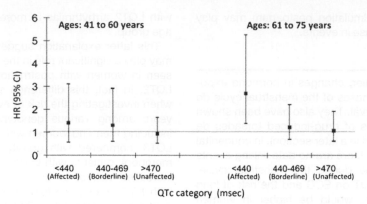

Fig. 6. Male versus female risk of aborted cardiac arrest (ACA) or death by QTc category and age group. Male versus female adjusted hazard ratio (HR) for ACA or death in each QTc category by age group is shown. Findings were adjusted for the following additional covariates: gender, time-dependent syncope less than 2 years previously and time-dependent syncope 2 to 10 years previously, and QTc duration (dichotomized at the upper quartile of each QTc category). Similar findings were obtained after further adjustment for time-dependent β-blocker therapy. CI, confidence interval. (*From* Goldenberg I, Moss AJ, Bradley J, et al. Long-QT syndrome after age 40. Circulation 2008;117(17):2198; with permission.)

This is a surprising finding because diabetes itself is associated with an increased QT interval.[55,56]

In contrast, development of coronary artery disease significantly increases the risk of syncope, aborted cardiac arrest, or sudden death in patients with LQTS.[57,58] In Sze and colleagues'[57] study, β-blocker use failed to reduce event rates in this group of patients. Furthermore, QTc and gender did not significantly affect the risk of events. The investigators suggest that myocardial disease and remodeling associated with ischemic heart disease may increase the risk of early afterdepolarizations and the risk of torsades de pointes.

Mechanistic insight into this clinical phenomenon may come from the long QT rabbit model. In a recently presented abstract,[58] LQT1 rabbits were significantly more prone to ventricular arrhythmias post myocardial infarct. The cause of this increase in arrhythmias seemed to be the emergence of new increase in repolarization heterogeneities in the noninfarcted left ventricular free wall adjacent to the infarct region. This heterogeneity was significantly increased compared with rabbits with LQT1 with a sham infarct or with rabbits without LQT1 that underwent the myocardial infarction protocol (**Fig. 7**). Further work may help decipher the mechanism for this new heterogeneity in repolarization after infarction. Thus, perhaps a genotype of LQTS may alter ventricular substrate and arrhythmias after myocardial infarction, rather than myocardial infarction altering the arrhythmia phenotype of LQTS.

It should be noted that exposure to bradycardia, electrolyte disorders, and QT-prolonging drugs increases with age. For patients with congenital LQTS, these conditions can represent the "second hit" on repolarization reserve that results in clinical events. The KCNE1 polymorphism D85 N, capable of causing LQTS with all its manifestations even in the absence of other predisposing factors,[59] is associated with clinical presentation later in life than some of the more severe LQTS mutations. In addition, D85 N is found in a disproportionately high number of patients presenting with torsades de pointes after receiving QT-prolonging drugs.[60] Thus, with increasing age and confounding medical conditions, patients with congenital LQTS may develop increased risk of clinical events due to acquired LQTS factors.

Acquired Long QT: Effects of Gender and Age

Women have a longer QT interval at baseline as we discussed earlier, likely stemming from the decrease in I_{Kr} from estrogen exposure and the lack of I_{Kr} potentiation from testosterone. As expected, these effects play a significant role in the development of drug-related acquired LQTS. Lehmann and colleagues[61] demonstrated that regardless of the dose of sotalol, ventricular repolarization as measured by the JT interval on ECG was significantly longer in women than in men.

More importantly, women have a higher risk of torsades de pointes in the presence of QT-prolonging drugs.[62] In fact, up to two-thirds of drug-related torsades de pointes occurs in women. Gender as a risk for drug-induced QT-related ventricular arrhythmias appears to be independent of weight adjusted dose or renal function.[63] Interestingly, in a meta-analysis including 332 reports

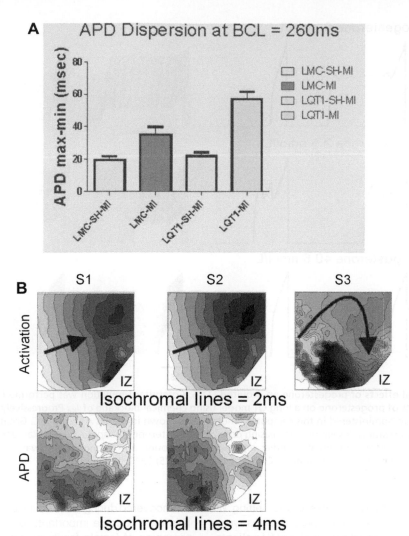

Fig. 7. Arrhythmogenesis and change in substrate in rabbits with LQT1 after myocardial infarction (MI). Data from a study of LQT1 transgenic rabbits and their littermate controls 3 weeks after either MI of the obtuse marginal of the left circumflex artery or sham procedure. The 4 groups are littermates with sham MI (LMC-SH-MI), littermates with true MI (LMC-MI), rabbits with LQT1 with sham MI (LQT1-SH-MI), and rabbits with LQT1 with true MI (LQT1-MI). Optical mapping of the left ventricular free wall of perfused whole hearts was performed. (*A*) Dispersion of action potential duration (APD) (maximum-minimum) in the left ventricular free wall in the 4 groups. The dispersion in LQT1-MI exceeds all other groups. (*B*) Reentry formation that ultimately leads to ventricular fibrillation in a perfused heart with programmed stimulation (S1-S2-S3 protocol). (*Adapted from* Ziv O, Schofield L, Chaves L, et al. Abstract 20881: increased peri-infarct calcium alternans underlies spontaneous VT and sudden death in LQT1 rabbits post myocardial infarction. Abstract presented at AHA November 2010. Circulation 2010;122(21 Meeting Abstracts):A20881; with permission.)

of drug-induced torsades de pointes, female gender as a risk for drug-induced torsades de pointes was independent of QTc. The steeper QT-RR relationship in women may explain this phenomenon.[22] Whereas the QT intervals of men and women are similar at shorter RR intervals, with bradycardia and longer RR intervals, QT prolongation is exaggerated in women. This may be because of the greater reliance on I_{Ks} for repolarization in women.

Acquired complete heart block, which occurs more commonly with advanced age, is a more extreme example of bradycardia. At least 2 large cases series have demonstrated that female gender is a potent risk factor for the development of torsades de pointes in patients presenting with acquired complete heart block. Kawasaki and colleagues[64] reported that between 1985 and 1992, 52% of hospital admissions for complete heart block were women, but 72% of the case

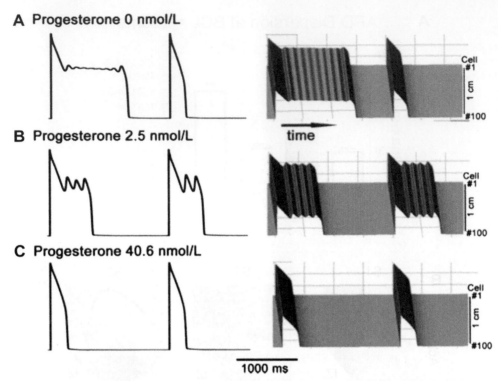

Fig. 8. Potential effects of progesterone on acquired LQTS. Computer simulation was performed illustrating the potential effects of progesterone on a long QT model using chemical blockade of I_{Kr}. Progressively larger doses of progesterone are administered in this computer simulation as shown in panels A through C. Greater reduction of early afterdepolarizations is seen with increasing doses of progesterone. (*Adapted from* Nakamura H, Kurokawa J, Bai CX, et al. Progesterone regulates cardiac repolarization through a nongenomic pathway: an in vitro patch-clamp and computational modeling study. Circulation 2007;116(25):2920; with permission.)

reports of torsades de pointes in the setting of heart block were in women. These findings were echoed by a more recent case series of 64 patients presenting with complete heart block to a single institution over a 3-year period. Of the 3 who had torsades de pointes on presentation, all were women exposed to bradycardia for more than 48 hours.[65,66] It is known from the rabbit model that prolonged exposure to bradycardia causes loss of repolarization reserve through downregulation of both I_{Ks} and I_{Kr}.[66,67] These changes are particularly hazardous in women, who have less repolarization reserve at baseline.

DIAGNOSTIC AND TREATMENT CONSIDERATIONS

Given the important role of hormones and the intricate relationship of gender and age in ventricular repolarization and susceptibility to LQTS-associated clinical events, we believe that consideration of these issues is justified in certain diagnostic or treatment scenarios. First, in a premenopausal woman, the longest QTc may be uncovered during the follicular phase of menses. This may become important, for example, in the screening of female family members of a patient with LQTS. Second, it is reasonable to take into consideration changes in the hormonal state (pregnancy, postpartum state, menopause) when making treatment recommendations to patients with LQTS. Third, the data support consideration of a patient's age and gender when considering treatment with QT-prolonging drugs. Even with comparable QTc, women are more susceptible than men to torsades de pointes when exposed to I_{Kr} blockade. Lower initial doses may be appropriate when starting older female patients on class III antiarrhythmic medications, for example.

Last, although research into age and gender effects on repolarization has helped clinicians make management decisions for patients with LQTS using current therapy, ultimately, further research into this aspect of the field may yield powerful new treatments. Computer simulations[25,68] suggest that exposure to progesterone may have antiarrhythmic effects in both drug-induced and congenital LQTS. In these studies, progesterone seemed to have a dose-related antiarrhythmic effect in reducing early afterdepolarizations and torsades de points (**Fig. 8**). More basic and clinical work will be needed to investigate this possible role for progesterone before any definitive recommendations can be made.

SUMMARY

Age and gender play a significant role in the determination of the QT interval via the complex effects of hormones on ventricular repolarization. These effects in turn significantly alter the clinical course of congenital LQTS. Changes in hormone exposure, especially withdrawal of hormone such as with the postpartum state and menopause, may significantly increase the risk of clinical events in some LQTS genotypes. A better understanding of these intricate relationships will undoubtedly be useful in the clinical management of these patients and may additionally spawn new treatments for LQTS-related arrhythmias.

REFERENCES

1. Guyton AC, Hall JE. Human physiology and mechanisms of disease. 6th edition. Philadelphia: Saunders; 1997.
2. Svechnikov K, Landreh L, Weisser J, et al. Origin, development and regulation of human Leydig cells. Horm Res Paediatr 2010;73(2):93–101.
3. Lewis K, Lee PA. Endocrinology of male puberty. Curr Opin Endocrinol Diabetes Obes 2009;16(1):5–9.
4. Araujo AB, Wittert GA. Endocrinology of the aging male. Best Pract Res Clin Endocrinol Metab 2011; 25(2):303–19.
5. Butler L, Santoro N. The reproductive endocrinology of the menopausal transition. Steroids 2011;76(7): 627–35.
6. Burger HG, Dudley EC, Robertson DM, et al. Hormonal changes in the menopause transition. Recent Prog Horm Res 2002;57:257–75.
7. Hale GE, Burger HG. Hormonal changes and biomarkers in late reproductive age, menopausal transition and menopause. Best Pract Res Clin Obstet Gynaecol 2009;23(1):7–23.
8. Landgren BM, Collins A, Csemiczky G, et al. Menopause transition: annual changes in serum hormonal patterns over the menstrual cycle in women during a nine-year period prior to menopause. J Clin Endocrinol Metab 2004;89(6):2763–9.
9. Challis JR. Endocrinology of late pregnancy and parturition. Int Rev Physiol 1980;22:277–324.
10. Fuchs AR, Fuchs F. Endocrinology of human parturition: a review. Br J Obstet Gynaecol 1984;91(10): 948–67.
11. Merri M, Moss AJ, Benhorin J, et al. Relation between ventricular repolarization duration and cardiac cycle length during 24-hour Holter recordings. Findings in normal patients and patients with long QT syndrome. Circulation 1992;85(5):1816–21.
12. Burke JH, Ehlert FA, Kruse JT, et al. Gender-specific differences in the QT interval and the effect of autonomic tone and menstrual cycle in healthy adults. Am J Cardiol 1997;79(2):178–81.
13. Rodriguez I, Kilborn MJ, Liu XK, et al. Drug-induced QT prolongation in women during the menstrual cycle. JAMA 2001;285(10):1322–6.
14. Kadish AH, Greenland P, Limacher MC, et al. Estrogen and progestin use and the QT interval in postmenopausal women. Ann Noninvasive Electrocardiol 2004;9(4):366–74.
15. Rautaharju PM, Zhou SH, Wong S, et al. Sex differences in the evolution of the electrocardiographic QT interval with age. Can J Cardiol 1992;8(7):690–5.
16. Macfarlane PW, McLaughlin SC, Devine B, et al. Effects of age, sex, and race on ECG interval measurements. J Electrocardiol 1994;27(Suppl): 14–9.
17. Pham TV, Rosen MR. Sex, hormones, and repolarization. Cardiovasc Res 2002;53(3):740–51.
18. Ramirez AH, Schildcrout JS, Blakemore DL, et al. Modulators of normal electrocardiographic intervals identified in a large electronic medical record. Heart Rhythm 2011;8(2):271–7.
19. Gambill CL, Wilkins ML, Haisty WK Jr, et al. T wave amplitudes in normal populations. Variation with ECG lead, sex, and age. J Electrocardiol 1995; 28(3):191–7.
20. Yang H, Elko P, Fromm BS, et al. Maximal ascending and descending slopes of the T wave in men and women. J Electrocardiol 1997;30(4):267–76.
21. Surawicz B. Puzzling gender repolarization gap. J Cardiovasc Electrophysiol 2001;12(5):613–5.
22. Stramba-Badiale M, Locati EH, Martinelli A, et al. Gender and the relationship between ventricular repolarization and cardiac cycle length during 24-h Holter recordings. Eur Heart J 1997;18(6):1000–6.
23. Genovesi S, Zaccaria D, Rossi E, et al. Effects of exercise training on heart rate and QT interval in healthy young individuals: are there gender differences? Europace 2007;9(1):55–60.
24. McGill HC Jr, Anselmo VC, Buchanan JM, et al. The heart is a target organ for androgen. Science 1980; 207(4432):775–7.
25. Nakamura H, Kurokawa J, Bai CX, et al. Progesterone regulates cardiac repolarization through a nongenomic pathway: an in vitro patch-clamp and computational modeling study. Circulation 2007;116(25): 2913–22.
26. McGill HC Jr, Sheridan PJ. Nuclear uptake of sex steroid hormones in the cardiovascular system of the baboon. Circ Res 1981;48(2):238–44.

27. Lin AL, McGill HC Jr, Shain SA. Hormone receptors of the baboon cardiovascular system. Biochemical characterization of myocardial cytoplasmic androgen receptors. Circ Res 1981;49(4):1010–6.

28. Kurokawa J, Tamagawa M, Harada N, et al. Acute effects of oestrogen on the guinea pig and human IKr channels and drug-induced prolongation of cardiac repolarization. J Physiol 2008;586(Pt 12): 2961–73.

29. Odening KE, Hyder O, Chaves L, et al. Pharmaco-genomics of anesthetic drugs in transgenic LQT1 and LQT2 rabbits reveal genotype-specific differential effects on cardiac repolarization. Am J Physiol Heart Circ Physiol 2008;295(6):H2264–72.

30. Brunner M, Peng X, Liu GX, et al. Mechanisms of cardiac arrhythmias and sudden death in transgenic rabbits with long QT syndrome. J Clin Invest 2008; 118(6):2246–59.

31. Kurokawa J, Suzuki T, Furukawa T. New aspects for the treatment of cardiac diseases based on the diversity of functional controls on cardiac muscles: acute effects of female hormones on cardiac ion channels and cardiac repolarization. J Pharmacol Sci 2009;109(3):334–40.

32. Ridley JM, Shuba YM, James AF, et al. Modulation by testosterone of an endogenous hERG potassium channel current. J Physiol Pharmacol 2008;59(3): 395–407.

33. Hara M, Danilo P Jr, Rosen MR. Effects of gonadal steroids on ventricular repolarization and on the response to E4031. J Pharmacol Exp Ther 1998; 285(3):1068–72.

34. Brouillette J, Trepanier-Boulay V, Fiset C. Effect of androgen deficiency on mouse ventricular repolarization. J Physiol 2003;546(Pt 2):403–13.

35. Er F, Gassanov N, Brandt MC, et al. Impact of dihydrotestosterone on L-type calcium channels in human ventricular cardiomyocytes. Endocr Res 2009;34(3):59–67.

36. Locati EH, Zareba W, Moss AJ, et al. Age- and sex-related differences in clinical manifestations in patients with congenital long-QT syndrome: findings from the International LQTS Registry. Circulation 1998;97(22):2237–44.

37. Wang PJ. Ventricular arrhythmias and sudden cardiac death. Malden (MA): Oxford: Blackwell Futura; 2008.

38. Priori SG, Schwartz PJ, Napolitano C, et al. Risk stratification in the long-QT syndrome. N Engl J Med 2003;348(19):1866–74.

39. Goldenberg I, Moss AJ, Peterson DR, et al. Risk factors for aborted cardiac arrest and sudden cardiac death in children with the congenital long-QT syndrome. Circulation 2008;117(17):2184–91.

40. Sauer AJ, Moss AJ, McNitt S, et al. Long QT syndrome in adults. J Am Coll Cardiol 2007;49(3): 329–37.

41. Wasserstrom JA, Kapur S, Jones S, et al. Characteristics of intracellular Ca2+ cycling in intact rat heart: a comparison of sex differences. Am J Physiol Heart Circ Physiol 2008;295(5):H1895–904.

42. Odening KE, Choi BR, Liu GX, et al. Abstract 15600: mechanisms of anti-arrhythmic effects of progesterone and pro-arrhythmic effects of estradiol in transgenic long qt type 2 rabbits. Circulation 2010; 122:A15600, 21-Meeting Abstracts.

43. Zareba W, Moss AJ, Locati EH, et al. Modulating effects of age and gender on the clinical course of long QT syndrome by genotype. J Am Coll Cardiol 2003;42(1):103–9.

44. Migdalovich D, Moss AJ, Lopes CM, et al. Mutation and gender-specific risk in type 2 long QT syndrome: implications for risk stratification for life-threatening cardiac events in patients with long QT syndrome. Heart Rhythm 2011;8(10):1537–43.

45. Roden DM, Balser JR. A plethora of mechanisms in the HERG-related long QT syndrome. Genetics meets electrophysiology. Cardiovasc Res 1999; 44(2):242–6.

46. Wei J, Wang DW, Alings M, et al. Congenital long-QT syndrome caused by a novel mutation in a conserved acidic domain of the cardiac Na+ channel. Circulation 1999;99(24):3165–71.

47. January CT, Gong Q, Zhou Z. Long QT syndrome: cellular basis and arrhythmia mechanism in LQT2. J Cardiovasc Electrophysiol 2000;11(12):1413–8.

48. Roden DM. Long QT syndrome: reduced repolarization reserve and the genetic link. J Intern Med 2006; 259(1):59–69.

49. Seth R, Moss AJ, McNitt S, et al. Long QT syndrome and pregnancy. J Am Coll Cardiol 2007;49(10): 1092–8.

50. Khositseth A, Tester DJ, Will ML, et al. Identification of a common genetic substrate underlying postpartum cardiac events in congenital long QT syndrome. Heart Rhythm 2004;1(1):60–4.

51. Antzelevitch C. Ionic, molecular, and cellular bases of QT-interval prolongation and torsade de pointes. Europace 2007;9(Suppl 4):iv4–15.

52. Buber J, Mathew J, Moss AJ, et al. Risk of recurrent cardiac events after onset of menopause in women with congenital long-QT syndrome types 1 and 2. Circulation 2011;123(24):2784–91.

53. Goldenberg I, Moss AJ, Bradley J, et al. Long-QT syndrome after age 40. Circulation 2008;117(17): 2192–201.

54. Ouellet G, Moss AJ, Jons C, et al. Influence of diabetes mellitus on outcome in patients over 40 years of age with the long QT syndrome. Am J Cardiol 2010;105(1):87–9.

55. Giunti S, Bruno G, Lillaz E, et al. Incidence and risk factors of prolonged QTc interval in type 1 diabetes: the EURODIAB prospective complications study. Diabetes Care 2007;30(8):2057–63.

56. Rutter MK, Viswanath S, McComb JM, et al. QT prolongation in patients with Type 2 diabetes and microalbuminuria. Clin Auton Res 2002;12(5):366–72.

57. Sze E, Moss AJ, Goldenberg I, et al. Long QT syndrome in patients over 40 years of age: increased risk for LQTS-related cardiac events in patients with coronary disease. Ann Noninvasive Electrocardiol 2008;13(4):327–31.

58. Ziv O, Schofield L, Chaves L, et al. Abstract 20881: increased peri-infarct calcium alternans underlies spontaneous VT and sudden death in LQT1 rabbits post myocardial infarction. Circulation 2010;122: A20881, 21 Meeting Abstracts.

59. Nishio Y, Makiyama T, Itoh H, et al. D85N, a KCNE1 polymorphism, is a disease-causing gene variant in long QT syndrome. J Am Coll Cardiol 2009;54(9): 812–9.

60. Paulussen AD, Gilissen RA, Armstrong M, et al. Genetic variations of KCNQ1, KCNH2, SCN5A, KCNE1, and KCNE2 in drug-induced long QT syndrome patients. J Mol Med (Berl) 2004;82(3): 182–8.

61. Lehmann MH, Hardy S, Archibald D, et al. JTc prolongation with d, l-sotalol in women versus men. Am J Cardiol 1999;83(3):354–9.

62. Lehmann MH, Hardy S, Archibald D, et al. Sex difference in risk of torsade de pointes with d, l-sotalol. Circulation 1996;94(10):2535–41.

63. Makkar RR, Fromm BS, Steinman RT, et al. Female gender as a risk factor for torsades de pointes associated with cardiovascular drugs. JAMA 1993; 270(21):2590–7.

64. Kawasaki R, Machado C, Reinoehl J, et al. Increased propensity of women to develop torsades de pointes during complete heart block. J Cardiovasc Electrophysiol 1995;6(11):1032–8.

65. Yiginer O, Kilicaslan F, Aparci M, et al. Advanced age, female gender and delay in pacemaker implantation may cause TdP in patients with complete atrioventricular block. Indian Pacing Electrophysiol J 2010;10(10):454–63.

66. Tsuji Y, Zicha S, Qi XY, et al. Potassium channel subunit remodeling in rabbits exposed to long-term bradycardia or tachycardia: discrete arrhythmogenic consequences related to differential delayed-rectifier changes. Circulation 2006;113(3):345–55.

67. Qi X, Yeh YH, Chartier D, et al. The calcium/calmodulin/kinase system and arrhythmogenic afterdepolarizations in bradycardia-related acquired long-QT syndrome. Circ Arrhythm Electrophysiol 2009;2(3): 295–304.

68. Furukawa T, Kurokawa J, Clancy CE. A combined approach using patch-clamp study and computer simulation study for understanding long QT Syndrome and TdP in Women. Curr Cardiol Rev 2008;4(4):244–50.

Risk Stratification in the Long QT Syndrome

Andrea Mazzanti, MD[a], Carlo Napolitano, MD, PhD[b],
Silvia G. Priori, MD, PhD[c,d,e],*

KEYWORDS

• Long QT syndrome • Sudden death • Risk stratification

Concrete advances have been taken in the past 55 years in the comprehension and management of inherited pathologies that predispose individuals to an increased risk of sudden cardiac death (SCD). Since the first observation by Jervell and Lange-Nielsen[1] of "four cases of deaf-mutism combined with a marked prolongation of the QT interval and a serious outcome," physicians and scientists worldwide have collaborated to make the long QT syndrome (LQTS) the most investigated inherited arrhythmogenic syndrome. Several registries that have collected thousands of patients have allowed the natural history of this syndrome to be defined,[2,3] which has an estimated prevalence of 1 in every 2000 live births.[4]

ß-Blockers (especially in the context of specific LQTS subtypes; **Fig. 1**) have shown their efficacy in protecting most patients from dangerous ventricular arrhythmias and have dramatically improved the natural history of the disease.[5,6] A minority of affected individuals, however, remain at risk despite antiadrenergic therapy,[6] and therefore it has become of paramount importance to identify these patients and direct them to alternative and more aggressive therapeutic strategies, including cardiac denervation and an implantable cardioverter-defibrillator (ICD). An appropriate risk stratification scheme is pivotal to preventing sudden death while avoiding overtreatment.

Risk stratification is an evolving concept that began from the observation of clinical parameters (history of symptoms, QT duration, age, gender) and subsequently integrated knowledge from molecular studies (gene-specific initially, and mutation-specific in a future perspective).[3] Currently, the concept of determining individual risk is based on a well-established framework of clinical and genetic characteristics. A history of aborted cardiac arrest or syncope is the best predictor for future events. In asymptomatic individuals, corrected QT duration (QTc, $\geq$500 ms) is a good indicator for risk stratification, especially when combined with demographic and genetic characteristics (age, gender, LQTS subtype).

This article presents detailed data regarding the risk predictors in LQTS.

CLINICAL RISK PARAMETERS
Symptoms

LQTS exposes patients to an increased risk of fatal (SCD) and nonfatal arrhythmic events that persist from an early age and progress almost unabated until adulthood.[3] The overall annual rate of SCD in patients with untreated LQTS is approximately 0.9%.[7]

Syncope is a frequent event in patients with LQTS, with an annual rate of approximately 5%

This work received no funding support.

Conflict of interest: Andrea Mazzanti receives consulting fees from Health in Code S.L. - Spain.

a Instituto de Investigación Biomédica de la Universidad de A Coruña (INIBIC), Instituto de Ciencias de la Salud, As Xubias s/n - 15006 A Coruña, Spain
b Division of Molecular Cardiology, Fondazione Salvatore Maugeri, Via Salvatore Maugeri, 4 - 27100 Pavia, Italy
c Molecular Cardiology, IRCCS Fondazione Salvatore Maugeri, Pavia, Italy
d Department of Molecular Medicine, University of Pavia, Pavia, Italy
e Cardiovascular Genetics Program, Leon H. Charney Division of Cardiology, NYU Langone Medical Center, New York, NY, USA
* Corresponding author. Molecular Cardiology, IRCCS Fondazione Salvatore Maugeri, Pavia, Italy.
E-mail address: spriori@fsm.it

Card Electrophysiol Clin 4 (2012) 53–60
doi:10.1016/j.ccep.2011.12.006
1877-9182/12/$ – see front matter © 2012 Published by Elsevier Inc.

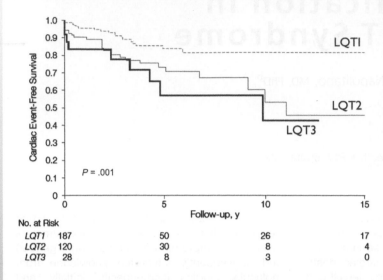

Fig. 1. Kaplan-Meier analysis of cumulative cardiac event-free survival in patients with genotyped LQTS receiving ß-blockers according to the genetic variant of the disease ($P = .001$ by the log-rank test). The definition of events included syncope, cardiac arrest, and sudden cardiac death. LQT1, long QT syndrome type 1; LQT2, long QT syndrome type 2; LQT3, long QT syndrome type 3. (*From* Priori SG, Napolitano C, Schwartz PJ, et al. Association of long QT syndrome loci and cardiac events among patients treated with beta-blockers. JAMA 2004;292:1343; with permission.)

in untreated patients, and some variability based on the underlying genetic defect.[3] Although probably not all syncopes observed in patients with LQTS are caused by arrhythmic events, a clinical history of a syncopal event is a strong predictor of adverse outcome.[7,8] A single syncopal event has been associated with a sixfold increase in the risk of subsequent SCD.[9] Jons and colleagues[10] showed that patients who experience multiple syncopes in the absence of ß-blocker treatment have twice the risk of experiencing a cardiac event compared with patients who have a single syncopal event (hazard ratio [HR], 1.8; $P<.001$). Additionally, this study showed that the occurrence of syncope during ß-blocker treatment is the most powerful predictor of subsequent life-threatening events (HR, 3.6; $P<.001$; **Fig. 2**) and indicates the need for more aggressive therapies. The risk of ß-blocker failure is apparently highest in young children and women.[10]

QT Interval Duration

Recording of 12-lead surface electrocardiogram and accurate measurement of QT interval corrected for heart rate (QTc) represent the basic evaluation for establishing the diagnosis of LQTS. As with most biologic parameters, the QT interval varies in relation to age and sex,[11] and is also modulated by fluctuations in heart rate or the autonomic tone. Besides being the hallmark of the syndrome, a prolonged QTc interval represents an effective indicator of risk in patients with LQTS.

That the probability of SCD and ventricular arrhythmias is strictly related to the magnitude of prolongation of the QT interval was originally shown in a study of the International Long QT Syndrome Registry in 1991.[7]

With the progressive importance that genetics has gained in the field, it seemed reasonable to reassess whether the introduction of genotype to the

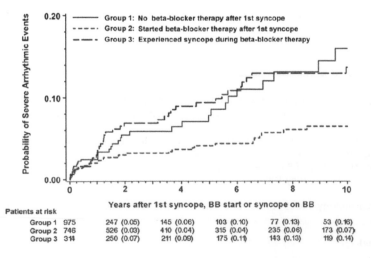

Fig. 2. The cumulative risk of severe arrhythmic events and ß-blocker (BB) therapy. The solid black line represents all patients after the first syncopal event until the start of BB therapy, and the red dashed line represents patients after the start of therapy. Patients with a syncopal event occurring while off BB therapy are represented by the purple dashed line. (*From* Jons C, Moss AJ, Goldenberg I, et al. Risk of fatal arrhythmic events in long QT syndrome patients after syncope. J Am Coll Cardiol 2010;55(8):785; with permission.)

risk stratification parameters would preserve a role for QT interval duration as an independent predictor of life-threatening arrhythmias and sudden death. In one such study, the authors[3] showed that the QT interval is influenced by the genetic locus (with average QTc being shorter in patients with LQTS type 1 [LQT1] than in those with other genotypes) and also confirmed that in a multivariate analysis, the QTc duration remains a predictor of cardiac events. Specifically, within each of the three more prevalent genetic variants of the disease (LQT1, LQTS type 2 [LQT2], and LQTS type 3 [LQT3]), patients with a QTc in the upper quartile present a risk of cardiac events that is five- to eightfold that of patients with a QTc duration in the first quartile (**Fig. 3**).

As a general rule, individuals with a QTc interval greater than 500 ms are at high risk for syncope or SCD, and require prophylactic therapy.[3]

Considering the critical role of QT interval duration in determining the probability of experiencing adverse events, an accurate measurement of the QT duration is clearly required. This apparently simple operation can be biased by both technical problems and the intrinsic polymorphic nature of the pathology. From a technical standpoint, it is important to standardize the method of measuring the QT interval. According to experts in the field and some elegant evidence from literature, the highest diagnostic and prognostic value in families with LQTS has been observed for QTc in leads II and V5 of 12-lead electrocardiograms. Thus, QT should be obtained in one of these leads, if measured in only one electrocardiogram lead.[12]

Another important aspect to consider when using the Bazett formula[13] to correct the QT interval is that the formula is linear for heart rates between 60 and 100 beats per minute. Finally, considering that the adaptation of the QT to changes in heart rate presents an hysteresis, avoiding QT measurement is recommended when the heart rate shows beat-by-beat instability. Whenever a stable heart rate is not possible to achieve (such as in atrial fibrillation), it is reasonable to select the recording showing less variability of the RR interval.[14]

Most patients with LQTS will have a QTc greater than 440 ms. However, some individuals may carry pathogenetic mutations without presenting a prolonged QT (incomplete penetrance). The prevalence of silent mutation carriers varies according to the genetic subtype and ranges from 36% in patients with LQT1 to 10% in those with LQT3.[3]

Additionally, even among patients with a definitive diagnosis of LQTS, Goldenberg and colleagues[15] found that the QTc interval is variable during repetitive electrocardiogram recordings, with a mean of 47 ± 40 ms: therefore, the risk stratification should not rely only on the baseline electrocardiogam. Periodic electrocardiograms at follow-up are required to promptly identify any change in QT that may occur over time.

As shown by Moss and colleagues[7] in 1991 and confirmed in a subsequent study by Barsheshet and colleagues,[16] increased resting heart rate is an independent predictor of life-threatening cardiac events in patients with LQT1.

Among the electrocardiogram parameters not yet validated, but still very interesting, clinical

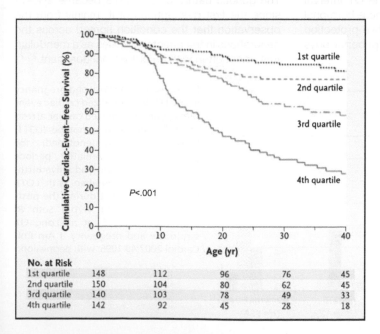

Fig. 3. Kaplan-Meier estimates of cumulative survival free of cardiac events among 580 patients from the International LQT Registry, according to the quartile of the QT interval corrected for heart rate (QTc). The four quartiles of QTc were as follows: first, ≤446 ms; second, 447–468 ms; third, 469–498 ms; and fourth, >498 ms. The difference among the quartiles was significant (P<.001). (*From* Priori SG, Schwartz PJ, Napolitano C, et al. Risk stratification in the long-QT syndrome. N Engl J Med 2003;348:1870; with permission.)

No. at Risk				
1st quartile	148	112	96	76	45
2nd quartile	150	104	80	62	45
3rd quartile	140	103	78	49	33
4th quartile	142	92	45	28	18

markers reflect heterogeneity of myocardial repolarization and could be related to an increased arrhythmic risk, including abnormal T-wave alternans, an increased T_{peak}–T_{end} interval, and dispersion of mechanical contraction time.[17]

Age and Gender

In early epidemiologic studies, an excess of affected women became apparent, representing 60% to 70% of patients with LQTS.[7] In the genetic era, this observation was placed in the context of an autosomal dominant pattern of inheritance and explained as a higher penetrance of the disease among women.[3] The reasons that make them more prone to respond to the presence of mutations in ion channels with prolongation of QT, and men more resistant to manifest the phenotype, remain a matter of debate.

One of the most appealing explanations for these gender differences in the manifestations of the disease has been attributed to the complex influences that sex hormones exert on the electric activity of the heart.[11,18] A collaborative study provided an alternative explanation for this predominance, showing an increased probability of maternal transmission of the LQTS-affected allele to daughters over sons.[19]

The possible relationship between female hormones and arrhythmic risk is supported by the evidence that a significant increase in the risk of cardiac events occurs in the 9-month postpartum period, mainly among women with an LQT2 mutation (**Fig. 4**).[20]

However, the evidence that androgens, and specifically testosterone, shorten the QT interval in boys after puberty suggests that these hormonal influences might account for a relative protection from life-threatening events in postpubertal boys and men with LQTS.[21]

A most important influence of gender is observed on the modulation that it exerts on the severity of the clinical manifestations.[21]

A recent analysis from the International LQTS Registry showed that during childhood, male sex is associated with a threefold increase in the risk of life-threatening cardiac events (**Fig. 5**).[8] This effect seems to be accentuated in families with LQT1.[3,8,21,22]

However, after puberty, an opposite trend has been observed, and women maintain a higher risk than men during adulthood. In an analysis of 812 patients with genotype-positive LQTS, Sauer and colleagues[23] found that women between ages 18 and 40 years show a higher risk (2.7-fold) and higher cumulative probability (11% vs 3%) of aborted cardiac arrest and SCD than men (**Fig. 6**).

After the age of 40 years, women still exhibit a significant higher arrhythmic risk than men,[23] which seems to counterbalance the increased male risk from acquired cardiovascular pathologies in the older age groups. Buber and colleagues[24] recently showed a genotype-specific association with the risk for cardiac events during the perimenopausal period, including a pronounced increase in the risk for arrhythmic events (mainly recurrent syncopes) among women with LQT2 and an opposite reduction in women with LQT1 (**Fig. 7**).

A partial exception to this comes from LQT3, in which men exhibit an increased risk of SCD across the lifespan.[3]

Genetic Risk Parameters

The genetic nature of the LQTS became evident since the first descriptions of it, mainly from the observation that the condition spread across the generations in the affected families as a mendelian trait, most often with an autosomal dominant,[25,26]

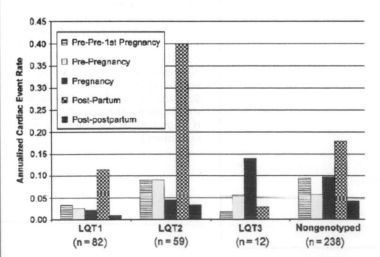

Fig. 4. Arrhythmic risk and pregnancy in the LQTS. Annualized cardiac event rates (syncope, aborted cardiac arrest, or LQTS death) by genotype (LQT1, LQT2, LQT3, nongenotyped) for defined pregnancy-related periods for 391 women who had a live birth. None of the 12 women with LQT3 had a cardiac event during the post-postpartum period. (*From* Seth R, Moss AJ, McNitt S, et al. Long QT syndrome and pregnancy. J Am Coll Cardiol 2007;49:1096; with permission.)

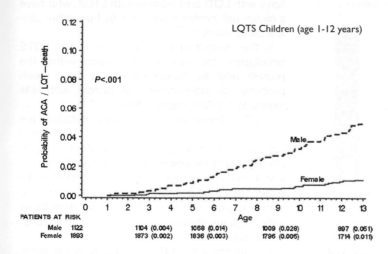

Fig. 5. Kaplan-Meier estimates of the probability of aborted cardiac arrest or sudden cardiac death in 3015 children between 1 and 12 years of age from the International LQT Registry, by gender (values in parentheses are event rates). (*From* Goldenberg I, Moss AJ, Peterson DR, et al. Risk factors for aborted cardiac arrest and sudden cardiac death in children with the congenital long-QT syndrome. Circulation 2008;117:2187; with permission.)

and rarely with an autosomal recessive, pattern of inheritance.[1] These intuitions have since been confirmed in the course of the "genetic revolution," initiated in the early 1990s,[27] leading to the discovery of the heterogeneous substrate for the LQTS and to the comprehension of its pathophysiology.

To date, mutations in at least 13 genes have been linked to an LQTS phenotype (both isolated or in the context of multiorgan syndromes), with hundreds of variants described and even more expected to emerge in parallel with the extensive use of new tools for massive sequencing (see article by Schulze-Bahr elsewhere in this issue). Despite this complexity, the three first described forms of LQTS (LQT1 and LQT2, originated from loss-of-function mutations in potassium channels *KCNQ1* and *KCNH2*; LQT3 with gain-of-

function mutation in sodium channel *SCN5A*) account for approximately 80% of all genetically confirmed cases[28] and are the most completely characterized.

Numerous genotype–phenotype correlations have been discovered to date, including genotype-suggestive electrocardiogram patterns and triggers for cardiac events, and genotype-based natural histories and responses to drugs.[28–32] The genetic test has become clinically available to physicians treating patients with LQTS, and has joined traditional risk factors as an independent prognostic determinant[33] for these patients. It has also been contemplated by specific guidelines.[28]

A gene-specific risk profile was the first to be attempted (**Fig. 8**)[3,34]; this approach has subsequently been redefined with more precision (mutation site and effect on the function of the

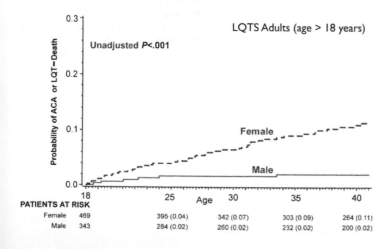

Fig. 6. Probability of aborted cardiac arrest (ACA) or sudden death after age 18 years, among 812 mutation-confirmed patients from the International LQT Registry, according to gender (unadjusted *P*<.001 by the log-rank test). (*From* Sauer AJ, Moss AJ, McNitt S, et al. Long QT syndrome in adults. J Am Coll Cardiol 2007;49:333; with permission.)

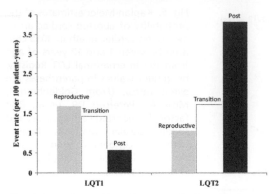

Rate of Cardiac Events by Menopausal Stages in LQT1 and LQT2 women

Fig. 7. Rate (per 100 patient-years) of cardiac events of any type (comprising syncope, aborted cardiac arrest, or sudden cardiac death) during follow-up among women with LQT1 and LQT2 by menopausal period. Event rates per 100 person-years among women with LQT1 and LQT2 were calculated by dividing the number of events during each menopausal period by the follow-up time in the same period and multiplying the result by 100. (*From* Buber J, Mathew J, Moss AJ, et al. Risk of recurrent cardiac events after onset of menopause in women with congenital long-QT syndrome types 1 and 2. Circulation 2011;123:2786; with permission.)

channel), and will reach a mutation-specific risk profile in the near future.

Compared with patients with the more common LQT1 and LQT2, those with LQT3 seem to have the highest mortality per event.[30] Exceptions are boys with LQTI and women with LTQ2, who have a higher risk profile independently from other clinical parameters.[22–24,35]

In the context of each of the two main LQTS genotypes, the mutation's location within the protein and its functional effects have been proposed as independent risk factors, with HRs similar to the QTc beyond 500 ms.[36,37]

In LQT1, transmembrane-located mutations are associated with a longer QTc and more frequent cardiac events than C-terminal mutations.[38] Additionally, LQT1 mutations with a dominant negative effect on the ion channel activity (ie, that provoke a reduction of >50% in its function) are associated with a greater risk of cardiac events than those with haploinsufficient behavior (ie, <50% functional reduction).[36]

In patients with LQT2, mutations in the pore-forming region (S5-loop-S6) of the *KCNH2* gene seem to have a greater risk of arrhythmic events than those with nonpore mutations.[37,39] A recent paper by Migdalovich and colleagues[40] found that the mutation site affected the risk of cardiac events in men with LQT2 (pore region at greater risk), whereas it is not relevant in women with LQT2, whose risk is high regardless of mutation location.

Besides an observed risk-stratifying class effect based on mutation type, location, and impact on cellular function, mutation-specific risk stratification has emerged for some discrete causative mutations (eg, A341V-*KCNQ1*, E1784K-*SCN5A*), and this approach will probably impact clinical

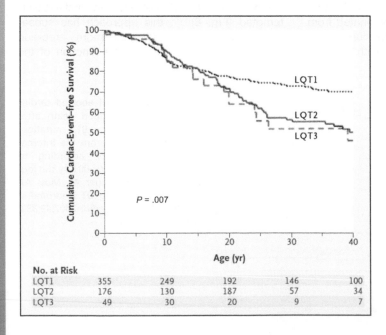

Fig. 8. Kaplan-Meier estimates of survival free of cardiac events among 580 patients from the International LQT Registry, according to the genetic locus of the mutation. The difference among the groups was significant ($P = .007$ by the log-rank test). (*From* Priori SG, Schwartz PJ, Napolitano C, et al. Risk stratification in the long-QT syndrome. N Engl J Med 2003;348:1869; with permission.)

No. at Risk				
LQT1	355	249	192	146	100
LQT2	176	130	187	57	34
LQT3	49	30	20	9	7

practice in the near future when the effect of a set of common mutations is better defined.[41,42]

Up to 4% to 11% of patients with genotyped LQTS may have a second pathogenic mutation in one of the LQTS-related genes and may have a more severe prognosis.[43–45] Therefore, a complete screening of the entire coding region of the three major LQTS genes (*KCNQ1*, *KCNH2*, and *SCN5A*) is advisable.[28]

SUMMARY

The long QT Syndrome is among the most prevalent arrhythmogenic conditions provoking a high risk of sudden death, throughout the life-span. Its hallmark is heterogeneity in genetic backgrounds, manifestations and prognosis. Beta-blockers effectively protect most patients, but a minority remain vulnerable despite drugs, requiring more aggressive therapies. A strategy for stratification, based on clinical and genetic parameters, is crucial to identify those at risk, while avoiding over-treatment. Symptoms (either cardiac arrest or syncope) are the strongest predictors for future events. In asymptomatic individuals, the QTc duration, together with demographic and genetic characteristics, are valid indicators of risk.

REFERENCES

1. Jervell A, Lange-Nielsen F. Congenital deaf-mutism, functional heart disease with prolongation of the Q-T interval, and sudden death. Am Heart J 1957;54: 59–68.
2. Schwartz PJ. The idiopathic long QT syndrome: the need for a prospective registry. Eur Heart J 1983; 4:529–31.
3. Priori SG, Schwartz PJ, Napolitano C, et al. Risk stratification in the long-QT syndrome. N Engl J Med 2003;348:1866–74.
4. Stramba-Badiale M, Crotti L, Goulene K, et al. Electrocardiographic and genetic screening for long QT syndrome: results from a prospective study on 44,596 neonates [abstract]. Circulation 2007; 116(Suppl II):II-377.
5. Schwartz PJ, Locati E. The idiopathic long QT syndrome: pathogenetic mechanisms and therapy. Eur Heart J 1985;6(Suppl D):103.
6. Priori SG, Napolitano C, Schwartz PJ, et al. Association of long QT syndrome loci and cardiac events among patients treated with beta-blockers. JAMA 2004;292:1341–4.
7. Moss AJ, Schwartz PJ, Crampton RS, et al. The long QT syndrome. Prospective longitudinal study of 328 families. Circulation 1991;84:1136–44.
8. Goldenberg I, Moss AJ, Peterson DR, et al. Risk factors for aborted cardiac arrest and sudden cardiac death in children with the congenital long-QT syndrome. Circulation 2008;117:2184–91.
9. Liu JF, Jons C, Moss AJ, et al. Risk factors for recurrent syncope and subsequent fatal or near-fatal events in children and adolescents with long QT syndrome. J Am Coll Cardiol 2011;57:941–50.
10. Jons C, Moss AJ, Goldenberg I, et al. Risk of fatal arrhythmic events in long QT syndrome patients after syncope. J Am Coll Cardiol 2010;55(8):783–8.
11. Surawicz B, Parikh SR. Differences between ventricular repolarization in men and women: description, mechanism and implications. Ann Noninvasive Electrocardiol 2003;8:333–40.
12. Mönnig G, Eckardt L, Wedekind H, et al. Electrocardiographic risk stratification in families with congenital long QT syndrome. Eur Heart J 2006;27: 2074–80.
13. Bazett HC. An analysis of time relations of the electrocardiograms. Heart 1920;7:353–70.
14. Lepeschkin E, Surawicz B. The measurement of the Q-T interval of the electrocardiogram. Circulation 1952;6:378–88.
15. Goldenberg I, Mathew J, Moss AJ, et al. Corrected QT variability in serial electrocardiograms in long QT syndrome: the importance of the maximum corrected QT for risk stratification. J Am Coll Cardiol 2006;48:1047–52.
16. Barsheshet A, Peterson DR, Moss AJ, et al. Genotype-specific QT correction for heart rate and the risk of life-threatening cardiac events in adolescents with congenital long-QT syndrome. Heart Rhythm 2011;8:1207–13.
17. Kaufman ES. Arrhythmic risk in congenital long QT syndrome. J Electrocardiol 2011;44:645–9.
18. Rivero A, Curtis AB. Sex differences in arrhythmias. Curr Opin Cardiol 2010;25:8–15.
19. Imboden M, Swan H, Denjoy I, et al. Female predominance and transmission distortion in the long-QT syndrome. N Engl J Med 2006;355:2744–51.
20. Seth R, Moss AJ, McNitt S, et al. Long QT syndrome and pregnancy. J Am Coll Cardiol 2007;49:1092–8.
21. Locati EH, Zareba W, Moss AJ, et al. Age- and sex-related differences in clinical manifestations in patients with congenital long-QT syndrome: findings from the International LQT Registry. Circulation 1998;97:2237–44.
22. Zareba W, Moss AJ, Locati EH, et al. Modulating effects of age and gender on the clinical course of long QT syndrome by genotype. J Am Coll Cardiol 2003;42:103–9.
23. Sauer AJ, Moss AJ, McNitt S, et al. Long QT syndrome in adults. J Am Coll Cardiol 2007;49: 329–37.
24. Buber J, Mathew J, Moss AJ, et al. Risk of recurrent cardiac events after onset of menopause in women

with congenital long-QT syndrome types 1 and 2. Circulation 2011;123:2784–91.

25. Romano C, Gemme G, Pongiglione R. Aritmie cardiache rare dell'età pediatrica. Clin Pediatr 1963; 45:656.

26. Ward OC. New familial cardiac syndrome in children. J Ir Med Assoc 1964;54:103.

27. Keating MT, Atkinson D, Dunn C, et al. Linkage of a cardiac arrhythmia, the long QT syndrome, and the Harvey ras-1 gene. Science 1991;252:704–6.

28. Ackerman MJ, Priori SG, Willems S, et al. HRS/EHRA expert consensus statement on the state of genetic testing for the channelopathies and cardiomyopathies. Europace 2011;13:1077–109.

29. Zhang L, Timothy KW, Vincent GM, et al. Spectrum of ST-T-wave patterns and repolarization parameters in congenital long-QT syndrome: ECG findings identify genotypes. Circulation 2000;102: 2849–55.

30. Schwartz PJ, Priori SG, Spazzolini C, et al. Genotype-phenotype correlation in the long-QT syndrome: gene-specific triggers for life-threatening arrhythmias. Circulation 2001;103:89–95.

31. Ackerman MJ. The long QT syndrome. Pediatr Rev 1998;19:232–8.

32. Choi G, Kopplin LJ, Tester DJ, et al. Spectrum and frequency of cardiac channel defects in swimming-triggered arrhythmia syndromes. Circulation 2004; 110:2119–24.

33. Schwartz PJ, Stramba-Badiale M, Crotti L, et al. Prevalence of the congenital long-QT syndrome. Circulation 2009;120:1761–7.

34. Zareba W, Moss AJ, Schwartz PJ, et al. Influence of the genotype on the clinical course of the long-QT syndrome. N Engl J Med 1998;339:960–5.

35. Goldenberg I, Moss AJ, Bradley J, et al. Long-QT syndrome after age 40. Circulation 2008;117: 2192–201.

36. Moss AJ, Shimizu W, Wilde AA, et al. Clinical aspects of type-1 long-QT syndrome by location, coding type, and biophysical function of mutations involving the KCNQ1 gene. Circulation 2007;115: 2481–9.

37. Shimizu W, Moss AJ, Wilde AA, et al. Genotype-phenotype aspects of type 2 long QT syndrome. J Am Coll Cardiol 2009;54:2052–62.

38. Shimizu W, Horie M, Ohno S, et al. Mutation site specific differences in arrhythmic risk and sensitivity to sympathetic stimulation in LQT1 form of congenital long QT syndrome: multicenter study in Japan. J Am Coll Cardiol 2004;44:117–25.

39. Moss AJ, Zareba W, Kaufman ES, et al. Increased risk of arrhythmic events in long-QT syndrome with mutations in the pore region of the human ether-a-go-go-related gene potassium channel. Circulation 2002;105:794–9.

40. Migdalovich D, Moss AJ, Lopes CM, et al. Mutation and gender-specific risk in type 2 long QT syndrome: implications for risk stratification for life-threatening cardiac events in patients with long QT syndrome. Heart Rhythm 2011;8:1537–43.

41. Crotti L, Spazzolini C, Schwartz PJ, et al. The common long-QT syndrome mutation KCNQ1/A341V causes unusually severe clinical manifestations in patients with different ethnic backgrounds: toward a mutation-specific risk stratification. Circulation 2007;116:2366–75.

42. Makita N, Behr E, Shimizu W, et al. The E1784K mutation in SCN5A is associated with mixed clinical phenotype of type 3 long QT syndrome. J Clin Invest 2008;118:2219–29.

43. Westenskow P, Splawski I, Timothy KW, et al. Compound mutations: a common cause of severe long-QT syndrome. Circulation 2004;109:1834–41.

44. Tester DJ, Will ML, Haglund CM, et al. Compendium of cardiac channel mutations in 541 consecutive unrelated patients referred for long QT syndrome genetic testing. Heart Rhythm 2005;2:507–17.

45. Itoh H, Shimizu W, Hayashi K, et al. Long QT syndrome with compound mutations is associated with a more severe phenotype: a Japanese multicenter study. Heart Rhythm 2010;7:1411–8.

Long QT Syndrome in the Very Young: Fetal Life Through Infancy

Andrew D. Blaufox, MD, FHRS

KEYWORDS

- Long QT syndrome • Infants • Neonates • Fetuses
- Outcome • Medical therapy • ICDs

Congenital long QT syndrome (LQTS) has recently been estimated to occur in approximately 1 in 2500 individuals.[1] Although LQTS is a genetic disorder, few patients will experience a cardiac event before the age of 1 year.[2] Those who do present during infancy, however, have a high rate of serious cardiac events, such as aborted cardiac arrest (ACA) or sudden cardiac death (SCD).[3,4] It is likely that many additional infants die of LQTS without the diagnosis ever being made, as LQTS may be responsible for approximately 10% of sudden infant death syndrome (SIDS) fatalities.[5] Thus, it is imperative that clinicians are aware of the historical and clinical findings associated with LQTS in the fetus, neonate, and infant to increase the likelihood that these children are diagnosed before they experience life-threatening symptoms. The need for early detection also raises questions regarding universal electrocardiogram (ECG) screening in neonates.[6] Although traditional beta-blocker therapy may be effective in infants who present without severe symptoms, beta-blocker therapy may not be as effective in those who present with severe symptoms.[2] Therefore, some of these infants will require more aggressive therapies, such as left cardiac sympathetic denervation or internal cardioverter-defibrillator (ICD) implantation. These strategies present new problems for caregivers, however, either because of limited data regarding their use in this specific population or because of practical considerations regarding their implementation in very small children. Because penetrance in LQTS is very low,[7] predicting which infants will be less likely to respond to beta-blockers will become increasingly more challenging as more of these children present as a result of screening (family or universal) before they are symptomatic.[8] While recognizing the anxiety such a diagnosis creates in a family,[9] caregivers must provide close follow-up with repeated education and stress the importance of compliance.

PRESENTATION

Timing of Presentation

Presentation has been reported to occur anytime before 1 year of age, including in fetuses, neonates, and older infants.[3,4] Reasons for presentation and symptoms experienced at presentation differ somewhat among these 3 subgroups. **Fig. 1** demonstrates 2:1 atrioventricular block (AVB) in a fetus referred for bradycardia who subsequently was diagnosed with LQTS on postnatal ECG (**Fig. 2**).

Modes of Presentation

Very young patients with LQTS most often present because of clinical suspicion based on cardiac events or screening because of family history.[2,3,8] Although every child born to a family with known LQTS should be evaluated for LQTS, the absence of LQTS in the family history does not rule out LQTS in any child. Children may be the first in their line to clinically manifest LQTS because they possess a de novo mutation[5] not seen in other family members or because they possess a

Electrophysiology, Division of Pediatric Cardiology, Department of Pediatrics, The Heart Center, The Steven and Alexandra Cohen Children's Medical Center of New York, North Shore–LIJ Hofstra School of Medicine, 269-01 76th Avenue, New Hyde Park, NY 11040, USA
E-mail address: Ablaufox@nshs.edu

Card Electrophysiol Clin 4 (2012) 61–73
doi:10.1016/j.ccep.2011.12.002
1877-9182/12/$ – see front matter © 2012 Elsevier Inc. All rights reserved.

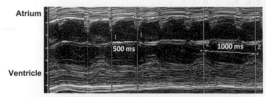

Fig. 1. Fetal echocardiogram in a patient with LQTS. This M-mode still is from a fetal echocardiogram performed for fetal bradycardia. It demonstrates 2:1 AV block. The atrial wall motion is shown above and the ventricular wall motion is shown below. The atrial rate is 120 bpm (cycle length = 500 msec) and the ventricular rate is 60 bpm (cycle length 1000 msec).

mutation carried by other family members, but these family members do not manifest LQTS because of the low penetrance of the mutation particular to that family.[7]

Clinical Features

Although very young children with LQTS may have no signs or symptoms at presentation, this group, as a whole, has a high rate of significant cardiac events.[3,4] These cardiac events include ACA, SCD, torsades de pointes (TdP), ventricular tachycardia (VT), syncope, seizures, sinus bradycardia, or AVB. The manner in which patients present is associated with their future outcome and response to therapy.

ACA/SCD
Presentation

In a Japanese nationwide survey, Horigome and colleagues[3] demonstrated that 7 (12%) of 58 children who presented with LQTS before the age of 1 year, presented with ACA or SCD. Garson and colleagues[4] showed that a higher proportion of children younger than 1 month presented with cardiac arrest than those who presented at an older age: 16% versus 7%, respectively (P<.05).

In a large LQTS Registry study, Spazzolini and colleagues[2] found the following risk factors associated with having ACA, SCD, or syncope in the first year of life (**Table 1**):

- QTc of 500 ms or longer
- Ventricular cycle length of 600 ms or longer
- Female gender.

Most patients who experienced cardiac events were either not genotyped or had negative genetic studies. This finding was also substantiated by Horigome and colleagues.[3] Although it is possible that the more severe symptoms seen in very young children are, in some cases, a result of rare novel mutations, the influence of genotype on presentation with ACA or SCD before the age of 1 year is not clear; however, SCN5A mutations have been identified in approximately 50% of the LQT mutations identified in large series of victims of SIDS.[5] This overrepresentation of SCN5A suggests an important role of SCN5A in the presentation of LQTS in very young children.

Prognosis

Patients who have experienced ACA before the age of 1 year are at significantly greater risk of experiencing future lethal or near lethal events (**Fig. 3**).[2] These patients have 23.4 times greater risk of experiencing ACA or SCD from ages 1 to 10 years than those who did not have ACA during

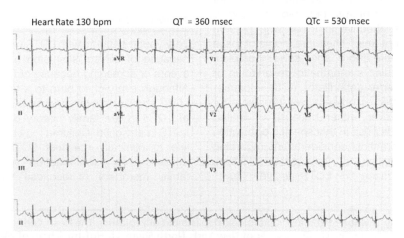

Fig. 2. Postnatal ECG in a patient with LQTS. This ECG was performed on the same patient as represented in **Fig. 1.** The patient is no longer bradycardic and no longer has AV block. The heart rate is 130 bpm and the QTc is 530 msec. The AV block and bradycardia did not recur after birth. This patient was found to have LQT2 and is doing well on beta blockade.

Table 1
Risk factors for sudden cardiac death, aborted cardiac arrest, or syncope in infants with long QT syndrome

Risk Factor	Hazard Ratio
QTc ≥500 ms	4.31
Ventricular cycle length ≥600 ms	2.38
Female gender	2.21
Genotype	NS

Abbreviation: NS, not significant.
  Data from Spazzolini DV, Mullally BS, Moss AJ, et al. Clinical implications for patients with long QT syndrome who experience a cardiac event during infancy. J Am Coll Cardiol 2009;54:832–7.

infancy.[2] The strength of this association with poor outcome is further illustrated by the fact that patients with ACA before the age of 1 year have 2.3 times greater risk for a second ACA or SCD from ages 1 to 10 years than those who experience their first ACA or SCD after age 1 year.[2] This risk of subsequent ACA or SCD after ACA or SCD in infancy was greater than that seen with a QTc of 500 ms or longer or gender and was still present after treatment with beta-blockers.[2]

TdP/VT
Presentation

TdP is a unique form of polymorphic ventricular tachycardia with changes in QRS axis and morphology that gives it the appearance of twisting around a central horizontal line. TdP may be transient and terminate in sinus rhythm or it may degenerate into ventricular fibrillation. TdP was noted in almost half of the Japanese children younger than 1 year reported by Horigome and colleagues,[3] including 7 of 18 fetuses, 15 of 31 neonates, and 5 of 9 older infants.[3] TdP/VT was proportionally more common in Japanese children younger than 1 year with LQT2 or LQT3 compared with those with LQT1 (10/11 vs 0/11, P<.001, and 5/6 vs 0/11, P<.005, respectively).[3]

Prognosis

Although there are limited data evaluating the association of TdP/VT experienced before the first year of life with future cardiac events in LQTS, TdP/VT is seen in patients with hemodynamic compromise or subsequent poor outcome, especially when it is associated with AVB.[10,11]

SYNCOPE
Presentation

Syncope is a clinical manifestation thought to be related to nonlethal ventricular arrhythmias significant and prolonged enough to result in hypoperfusion to the brain. Syncope is an unusual reported event in children younger than 1 year. Spazzolini and colleagues[2] found that 1% of patients with LQTS will present with syncope before the age of 1 year and Horigome and colleagues[3] found that syncope occurred in 5 of 31 neonates and 0 of 9 older infants. Syncope is difficult to detect in this

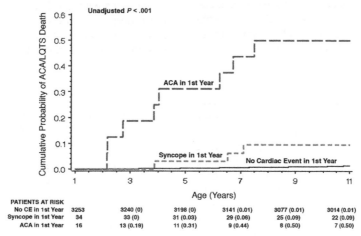

Fig. 3. Cumulative probability of ACA/LQTS-related death. The cumulative probability of aborted cardiac arrest/ LQTS-related death during ages 1 to 10 years is significantly greater in those who suffered ACA in the first year of life compared with those who had syncope in the first year of life or those who had no cardiac events in the first year of life. CE, cardiac event. (*From* Spazzolini DV, Mullally BS, Moss AJ, et al. Clinical implications for patients with long QT syndrome who experience a cardiac event during infancy. J Am Coll Cardiol 2009;54:832–7; with permission.)

age group because of the large amount of time these patients spend sleeping or laying in their cribs. Therefore, the incidence of syncope is likely to be underreported in children younger than 1 year.

Prognosis

Although syncope is not a surrogate for ACA or SCD, it is most commonly reported as a significant cardiac event with these 2 lethal or near lethal events in most large LQTS Registry studies.[12,13] In studies of older children, syncope has been shown to be associated with a greater likelihood of future ACA or SCD, especially if it is repetitive or occurs while the patient is being treated with beta-blockers[14,15]; however, such an association in children younger than 1 year has not been established by the data in the literature.[2] Interpretation of that data must be undertaken cautiously, as the incidence of syncope in this population is likely underreported and any associations, or lack of associations, between syncope and ACA or SCD may, therefore, not be accurately established.

SEIZURES
Presentation

Like syncope, seizures may be caused by ventricular arrhythmias significant enough to result in hypoperfusion to the brain. The reporting of seizures in very young children is relatively rare. Horigome and colleagues[3] reported seizures in 5 of 31 neonates and 0 of 9 older infants.

Prognosis

Although there are limited data regarding association of seizures with outcome in LQTS, it is probably prudent to view seizures in the same light as syncope until such data are reported.

BRADYCARDIA
Presentation

Sinus bradycardia is a common finding in children younger than 1 year with LQTS.[3,16,17] Horigome and colleagues[3] reported sinus bradycardia in 15 of 18 fetuses, 17 of 31 neonates, and 5 of 9 older infants. The bradycardia in children with LQTS persists until they are approximately 3 years old, after which there is no difference in heart rate between children with LQTS and those without LQTS.[17] Limited data from a study by Lupoglazoff and colleagues,[10] in which 23 neonates with LQTS and ventricular rates slower than 110 boats per minute (bpm) were identified, showed an association between sinus bradycardia and KCNQ1 mutations.

Prognosis

Profound bradycardia can be associated with pause-dependent ventricular arrhythmias. Spazzolini and colleagues[2] showed that having a heart rate slower than 100 bpm was associated with a 2.38 times greater risk of having ACA or SCD in the first year of life; however, this study did not stipulate whether the etiology of the bradycardia was sinus bradycardia or AVB.

AVB
Presentation

AVB is thought to occur in approximately 5% of children with LQTS,[4] but appears to be more common in those presenting when younger than 1 year. Horigome and colleagues[3] reported that AVB was seen in 8 of 18 fetuses, 10 of 31 neonates, and 5 of 9 older infants with LQTS. AVB in LQTS is usually AVB with 2:1 AV conduction.[4,10,11,18] This 2:1 AVB in LQTS is thought to be a functional block-related profound QTc prolongation rather than intrinsic disease of the conduction system and is caused by antegrade impulses of sinus rhythm terminating at the ventricle, as they arrive during periods of prolonged refractoriness.[11,18] The subsequent impulse can depolarize the ventricle, which is no longer refractory once repolarization has had time to occur (**Fig. 4**).

AVB may occur more frequently in females than males and may be more common in patients with a negative family history.[11]

AVB seems to be less common in LQT1 than LQT2.[3,10] Lupoglazoff and colleagues[10] evaluated 23 neonates with LQTS, of whom 15 had 2:1 AVB and 8 had sinus bradycardia. All 8 of those with sinus bradycardia had a KNCQ1 mutation, whereas 9 of 10 patients with 2:1 AVB who

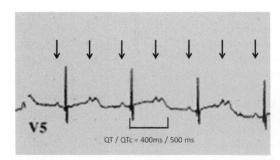

Fig. 4. AVB on ECG. This rhythm strip demonstrates 2:1 AVB in a patient with LQTS. The "p" waves are demarcated by arrows. The atrial rate is twice the ventricular rate. The QTc = 500 msec and the peak of the "T" wave occurs later than the nonconducted "p" wave.

underwent genetic testing had a HERG mutation, of whom one also had a KCNQ1 mutation. Although the sample size was smaller in Horigome and colleagues' study,[3] the proportion of patients with AVB was nearly significantly greater among those with LQT3 than those with LQT1 (5/6 vs 1/11, P = .068).

Prognosis

Patients with AVB tend to be more symptomatic on presentation than those without AVB.[10,11] It is seen in patients with TdP. Early studies indicated that the mortality of patients with LQTS with 2:1 AVB is very high; reaching 50% at 6 months and 67% at 2 years.[11] Fatal events are associated with VT, which are often pause dependent.[11] This is not surprising considering that a markedly prolonged QT interval is often seen in patients with AVB and that a QTc longer than 500 msec is independently associated with an increased risk of significant cardiac events.[19] Spazzolini and colleagues[2] found that a heart rate slower than 100 bpm was associated with a greater risk for SCD or ACA before the age of 1. Although this study did not comment on the etiology of this bradycardia, other studies have demonstrated that patients with LQTS with AVB tend to be more symptomatic than those with sinus bradycardia.[10] The prognosis of patients with LQTS with 2:1 AVB has improved recently with more prompt detection and interventions, as discussed in more detail in the treatment section later in this article.[10,18]

SIDS

In 2004, an expert panel defined SIDS as "…the sudden unexpected death of an infant <1 year of age, with onset of the fatal episode apparently occurring during sleep, that remains unexplained after a thorough investigation, including performance of a complete autopsy and review of the circumstances of death and the clinical history."[20] There were approximately 2100 SIDS cases in the United States in 2004, making it the third leading cause of infant mortality at a rate of 51 deaths per 100,000 live births.[21]

It is likely that the etiology of SIDS is multifactorial.[5] Commonly associated factors include maternal socioeconomic factors, maternal prenatal care, maternal smoking, infant gender, infant size, infant gestational age, and sleep position, among others.[22] The association between LQTS and SIDS was raised 35 years ago and a clear link between the 2 disorders was demonstrated in 1998.[23]

In a nearly 2-decade effort, Schwartz and colleagues[24] reviewed the ECGs of 24 victims of SIDS as well as a random sample of nearly 10,000 survivors. ECGs were performed on the third or fourth day of life to avoid the QTc variation that commonly occurs in the first 2 days of life.[25] They found that the victims of SIDS had a significantly longer QTc interval than those who survived (435 msec ± 45 msec vs 400 msec ± 20 msec, P<.01) and that neonates having a QTc greater than 440 msec (2 SDs above the mean for survivors) was associated with an odds ratio 41.3 for SIDS death.[24] Although this odds ratio is impressive and greater than that reported for other environmental and maternal factors,[26] the relative risk of SIDS associated with a prolonged QTc has not been directly compared with these environmental and maternal factors in the same population. Regardless, this study clearly demonstrated an association between SIDS and LQTS.

Shortly after this association was established, studies demonstrated a molecular link between LQTS and SIDS when postmortem analyses uncovered KVLQT1 and SCN5A mutations in several victims of SIDS.[27,28] In 2007, molecular screening of 7 LQTS genes was performed on a large cohort of Norwegian victims of SIDS. After subsequent functional analyses of these mutations, it was determined that 9.5% of the victims carried an LQTS mutation or rare variant that likely contributed to the death.[5] The manner in which these variants were thought to contribute to death fell into 3 categories: (1) the mutations by themselves caused marked channel dysfunction, (2) mutations caused marked channel dysfunction under specific environmental conditions, or (3) victims could possess multiple common variants that amplify any of the relatively minor deleterious effects seen when only one variant is present.

There are several additional interesting findings regarding the types of mutations that were found. SCN5A mutations were disproportionately overrepresented, such that most of the variants identified were in SCN5A in contrast to the observation that fewer than 10% of LQTS cases in the general population are associated with SCN5A mutations.[5] This suggests that SCN5A mutations may be more lethal in this very young population. The reasons for this are unknown. Another interesting finding was that a significant number of the variants found in the victims of SIDS were de novo variants not found in older populations. Perhaps the lethal nature of these mutations explains why they are not perpetuated to future generations and implies that screening for LQTS to prevent SIDS based on family history may be significantly limited.

To measure the scope of the impact of LQTS-related SIDS deaths, it would be illustrative to compare it to the problem of SCD in the young athlete, which is a tremendous issue of public concern. The incidence of SCD in young athletes is approximately 0.5 per 100,000 per year, accounting for approximately 75 deaths per year in the United States.[29] If the results of Arnestad and colleagues' study[5] are applied to the United States, more infants die of unrecognized LQTS each year, approximately 200. Considering that only 7 of the now-known 13 genes that cause LQTS were tested in Arnestad and colleagues' study,[5] as well as the fact that mutations are not found in approximately 15% of patients with LQTS, it is likely that additional SIDS deaths are related to LQTS.

DIAGNOSIS/WORKUP

The workup for LQTS in the very young will depend on his or her age of presentation, whether or not patients present with symptoms, and if there is an established preexisting family history of LQTS. In addition, workup of LQTS in those patients who have SCD will be somewhat different from others. Several scores have been developed to establish the diagnosis of LQTS,[30] but their accuracy has been called into question, particularly when evaluating nonprobands in a family with known LQTS.[31] There are few data regarding the validity of these systems in very young children. Workup for these children may include the following: thorough family history, ECG, Holter monitor, and genetic testing. In addition, a differential diagnosis list should be considered (**Table 2**).

Family History

An established diagnosis of LQTS in the child's family raises the suspicion that the child has LQTS, particularly if the child is severely symptomatic. As stated previously, however, an absent family history of LQTS/SCD cannot rule out this diagnosis in symptomatic or asymptomatic children. These children may be the first in their line to clinically manifest LQTS because they possess a de novo mutation[5] not seen in other family members or because they possess a mutation carried by other family members, but these family members do not manifest LQTS because of the low penetrance of the mutation particular to that family.[7]

In addition, the diagnosis of LQTS may not be realized despite family members being symptomatic because these symptoms are attributed to other diagnoses or simply have not been associated with LQTS. For instance, syncope related to undiagnosed LQTS is often classified as vasovagal and seizures are often attributed to intrinsic central nervous system disease. The etiology of SCD in a young family member must, likewise, be scrutinized, and every effort must be taken to obtain clear documentation of the cause of death. For example, the term "heart attack" is used liberally and does not provide definitive proof that the family member died of coronary artery disease rather than LQTS.

ECG

The mainstay of diagnosing LQTS is the ECG, where the QTc can be directly measured and T-wave morphology can be evaluated. Although the QTc can also be measured in utero with fetal electrocardiography,[32] the postnatal ECG is the more established method. Although a great deal of attention has been focused on the length of the QTc, it must also be remembered that patients

Table 2
Differential diagnosis for symptoms related to long QT syndrome and for prolongation of the QTc

Symptom/Sign	Differential Diagnosis
ACA	SIDS, CHD, metabolic disease, Brugada syndrome, congenital AVB
TdP	Electrolyte imbalance (hypokalemia, hypocalcemia, hypomagnesemia)
Syncope	Epilepsy, congenital AVB, stroke
Seizures	Epilepsy, stroke, metabolic disease, sepsis
AVB	Congenital AVB ($\pm$ maternal lupus)
Sustained Bradycardia	Hypothyroidism, increased CNS pressure, blocked atrial bigeminy
Prolonged QTc	Prolonged QTc of perinatal period, electrolyte imbalance (hypokalemia, hypocalcemia, hypomagnesemia), thyroid dysfunction, drugs, hypoxia, CNS abnormalities, maternal anti-Ro/SSA antibodies

Abbreviations: ACA, acute cardiac arrest; AVB, atrioventricular block; CHD, congenital heart disease; CNS, central nervous system; SIDS, sudden infant death syndrome; TdP, Torsades de Pointes.

with LQTS often have abnormal-appearing T waves.[33] In addition to performing ECGs on any child suspected of having LQTS, ECGs should also be performed on all immediate family members of any child newly diagnosed with LQTS, so as to provide further evidence for the diagnosis in the proband as well as to make the diagnosis in additional family members when that diagnosis had not been previously established in the family.

The ECG will also be helpful in documenting whether sinus bradycardia or AVB exist.

MEASURING THE QTc

Although very young children carrying genetic mutations for LQTS may not have prolonged QT intervals, 440 msec has been established as a threshold value for raising suspicion for the diagnosis of LQTS and prompting further evaluation for LQTS, particularly if the child has had severe associated symptoms or a family history of LQTS already exists.[4] It should also be recognized that a QTc longer than 440 msec may not be diagnostic of LQTS. The reasons for this are as follows:

1. There may be other causes of QTc prolongation (see **Table 2**).
2. There are inherent errors in QTc measurement.
3. The QTc may vary throughout one's life.
4. The QTc changes in the perinatal period.

Errors in QTc Measurement

Because the QT interval changes with heart rate, methods have been developed to correct the QT interval for heart rate. The Bazett method is most commonly used. The Bazett method may falsely prolong the QTc at very high heart rates and falsely shorten the QTc at very low heart rates.[34] In addition, the interobserver reliability of QTc measurements based on a single QTc measurement is low and it is suggested that an average of 3 independent measures provides the most reliable QTc measurement.[35]

Variation in QTc Throughout Life

Goldenberg and colleagues[36] demonstrated that there is considerable variability in QTc measurements in serial follow-up ECGs performed in patients with LQTS. The difference between the minimum and maximum QTc on serial ECGs was 47 ± 40 msec. Therefore, a child may have a normal QTc on one ECG, but may have an abnormal one on a subsequent ECG and visa versa.

Perinatal Changes in the QTc

The QTc may be prolonged in the first 2 days of life.[25] Therefore, the timing of the QTc measurement is of critical importance.

UNIVERSAL ECG SCREENING

The potential for LQTS to be undiagnosed in neonates who are susceptible for life-threatening symptoms or death is realized by the fact that approximately 10% of victims of SIDS may die from LQTS-related arrhythmias.[5] Although some patients will continue to have severe symptoms and die after LQTS is diagnosed,[2] it is likely that early recognition of LQTS and prompt therapeutic intervention will save many lives. This is why recognition of the signs and symptoms of LQTS, described previously, is critical. Because many of these children are likely to be asymptomatic in the perinatal period, many will not be diagnosed through standard practices and procedures, however. Therefore, the question of universal ECG screening is a valid topic of debate.

Although there is a great potential for LQTS to be diagnosed by ECG screening,[37] the institution of such a program is highly controversial.[6] Quaglini and colleagues[37] and others have demonstrated that neonatal ECG screening for LQTS is cost-effective, with estimates of approximately $16,500 to $18,500 per year of life saved or approximately $1.1 to $1.3 million for a 70-year life. Although the impact on detecting LQTS may even be greater than that noted for similar screening programs to prevent SCD in young athletes, the burden to the health system will likely be just as large. In an editorial letter in response to Quaglini and colleagues'[37] study, Van Hare and colleagues[38] argue that, given an incidence of LQTS of 1 in 2500, positive test rate of 1%, and a sensitivity of 80% for a QTc longer than 470 ms would yield a predictive value of 3%. In the United States, this would mean that approximately 1280 neonates with LQTS would be detected of 40,000 with positive tests. This would result in anxiety, further testing, and potential treatment of many thousands of children at no risk. Because of similar concerns, the American Heart Association recently made a statement indicating that ECG screening for 10,000,000 athletes would be cost-prohibitive and not recommended for the United States.[39] Although the estimated number of children screened for neonatal LQTS may be 40% of the number screened for athletics, the total costs would still be substantial. In addition to the financial issues, there would be many practical issues regarding neonatal ECG screening, including the timing of screening, considering that the QTc may be prolonged during the first week of life in children who do not have LQTS. In a survey study by Chang and colleagues,[6] half of the responding pediatric cardiologists felt that universal ECG screening could detect LQTS, only 31% felt that it could reduce the incidence of SIDS, and only 11% felt universal screening should be mandated. Further debate of this topic is encouraged.

Holter Monitor/Telemetry

Twenty-four-hour rhythm monitoring in the form of a Holter monitor for outpatients or telemetry for inpatients can be a useful adjunct in documenting the following supporting evidence for the diagnosis of LQTS and/or rhythms that may require more prompt intervention:

- AVB
- TdP
- Sustained sinus bradycardia
- T-wave alternans.

Genetic Testing

Genetic testing is extremely important in confirming the diagnosis in any child with a positive family history of LQTS and can also be helpful in establishing the diagnosis in children without a preexisting family history of LQTS. The predictive value of genetic testing in an individual depends on whether the genotype in that individual's family has already been determined.

Once the genotype in a family is established, genetic testing is a reliable method for determining if additional family members possess the family mutation or not. There should not be any delay in testing very young children if their familial mutation is already established, particularly if the clinical picture is not obvious. The results of this test will have a large impact on determining if therapy should be started, continued, or stopped.

In patients in whom a familial diagnosis or genotype is not established, genetic testing can confirm the diagnosis if the test is positive, but may not be helpful if the test is negative, as the negative predictive value of genetic testing of a proband with phenotypic LQTS is approximately 72%.[40] In addition, when the familial genotype is not known, testing the proband will provide specific information that may have a great impact on management strategy. For instance, finding an SCN5A mutation may prompt the use of sodium channel blockers, particularly if beta-blockers are ineffective.

In addition, LQTS must be considered in any child who suffers an SCD so as to provide answers for the child's family and to provide a basis of screening other family members. If SCD occurs before a diagnostic ECG is performed in a child without a family history, a postmortem genetic analysis can be accomplished to help provide these answers.[5,28]

Stepwise Workup

Recognizing that ECGs may be performed in the first few days of life for a variety of reasons, the European Society of Cardiology created a task force to provide guidelines for the interpretation of the neonatal ECG.[41] The logic of this plan can be applied to older infants, as indicated as follows in italic:

- If the first ECG performed in the first week of life shows a QTc longer than 440 msec,
  - a thorough family history should be taken with a focus on established LQTS, SCD, and possible clues to missed diagnoses stated previously.
  - second ECG should be performed a few days following the first.
  - If the second ECG is normal:
    - ... and the first QTc was 470 msec or shorter, dismiss the case.
    - ... and the first QTc was 470 msec or longer, plan a third ECG in 1 to 2 months.
  - If the second ECG shows a QTc between 440 msec and 470 msec (or if the first ECG in an older infant shows a QTc between 440 msec and 470 msec):
    - thorough family history should be taken with a focus on established LQTS, SCD, and possible clues to missed diagnoses stated previously.
    - other causes of QTc prolongation should be investigated.
    - For those without a family history of LQTS:
      - a Holter monitor should be obtained.
      - ECGs should be periodically reevaluated throughout the first year of life.
    - For those with a positive family history of LQTS:
      - a Holter monitor should be considered.
      - genetic testing should be performed.
      - initiation of medical therapy should be considered.
  - If the second ECG shows a QTc between 470 msec and 500 msec (or if the first ECG in an older infant shows a QTc between 470 msec and 500 msec):

- *a thorough family history should be taken with a focus on established LQTS, SCD, and possible clues to missed diagnoses stated previously.*
- other causes of QTc prolongation should be investigated.
- For those without a family history of LQTS:
  - a Holter monitor should be obtained.
  - ECGs should be periodically reevaluated throughout the first year of life.
  - medical therapy should be considered.
- For those with a positive family history of LQTS:
  - an additional ECG should be planned within 1 month.
  - a Holter monitor should be considered.
  - genetic testing should be performed.
  - medical therapy should be initiated.
- If the QTc normalizes over the next few months and testing does not confirm the diagnosis of LQTS, withdrawal of therapy can be considered.
  - If the second QTc is 500 msec or longer (*or if the first ECG in an older infant shows a QTc of 500 msec or longer*):
    - *a thorough family history should be taken with a focus on established LQTS, SCD, and possible clues to missed diagnoses stated previously.*
    - the child is likely to be affected and symptomatic.
    - all diagnostic testing stated previously should be performed.
    - the child should be treated.

TREATMENT

Treatment of LQTS in very young children can be challenging because the children may not respond as well to traditional therapy[2,42] and evidence for alternatives is lacking or practical considerations limit the implementation of these alternatives in small children.

Beta-Blockers

Beta-blockers have been established as the first line of medical therapy for LQTS, as they are usually well tolerated and have been shown to significantly reduce the rate of cardiac events in large LQTS Registry studies.[13] The effectiveness of beta-blockers in treating LQTS in children was questioned by Priori and colleagues,[42] who showed that beta-blockers were less effective in

preventing subsequent cardiac events, defined as syncope, TdP, VT, ACA, or SCD, in patients who experienced their first pretherapy cardiac event before the age of 7 years. When the analysis was limited to ACA and SCD, however, subsequent studies have demonstrated that beta-blockers are very effective in reducing the risk of ACA or SCD in the pediatric population taken as a whole.[15,43] Liu and colleagues[43] demonstrated that beta-blockers reduce the risk of subsequent ACA or SCD by more than 70% in children aged from birth to 20 years, even if they have recurrent syncope. Goldenberg and colleagues[15] examined children 1 to 12 years old and showed that the efficacy of beta-blockers was most pronounced if the patient recently experienced syncope within 2 years of the study but the effect was significantly less pronounced if syncope occurred remotely. Although Goldenberg and colleagues[15] did not look at children younger than 1, the number of very young children in Priori and colleagues'[42] and Liu and colleagues'[43] studies were relatively small and the effect of beta-blockers in very young children was not independently evaluated.

Spazzolini and colleagues[2] evaluated 212 patients with LQTS who had an ECG performed before 1 year of age and showed that beta-blockers are not effective in many very young children with LQTS. In this study, 4 of 20 children who died during infancy had been treated with beta-blockers and beta-blockers did not reduce the risk of subsequent ACA or SCD between 1 and 10 years of age in children who experienced remote syncope or who had ACA during infancy. Although beta-blockers are known to be less effective in LQT3 than LQT 1 or 2,[42] most of the very young children in this study were not genotyped and very few were known to be diagnosed with LQT3. Thus, there is no evidence that Spazzolini and colleagues'[2] findings can be attributed to a high proportion of infants with LQT3 in the study population. Regardless of the reason, alternate treatment strategies may be necessary to effectively treat some very young children.

Despite this, beta-blockers should be instituted for most very young children. Although they may not be effective in some, they are likely to be effective in those with less severe symptoms or those without symptoms.[15,43] This also appears to be true for siblings of patients who have died related to LQTS.[44] Although these siblings are more likely to be treated aggressively, having a sibling who died does not make the living sibling more likely to have an ACA or SCD.[44] It may be very difficult to convince parents of this fact, so the risks related to alternate therapies must be appreciated and fully explained to the family before proceeding with alternate therapies for a child without severe symptoms.

Sodium Channel Blockers

Sodium channel blockers have been shown to effectively reduce cardiac events in LQTS,[45] including children or fetuses.[46,47] Cuneo and colleagues[47] described the transplacental treatment of TdP with continuous maternal infusions of lidocaine in a fetus with LQTS and a QTc longer than 600 msec diagnosed by fetal magnetocardiography. The TdP was successfully controlled by lidocaine and the child was started on mexiletine in the postnatal period. Ten Harkel and colleagues[46] described a neonate with LQT3 whose ICD discharges subsided after increased dosing of flecainide resulted in adequate serum levels. Although these examples of the use of sodium channel blockers for LQT3 are encouraging, the data on their safety and efficacy in this population are very limited; however, it seems reasonable that sodium channel blockers should be considered for any very young child who is severely symptomatic of LQT3 and that these children should be followed closely to monitor for Brugada-like changes on the ECG, as well as continued symptoms that may require additional therapies.

Pacemakers

As mentioned earlier, bradycardia and 2:1 AVB have been associated with a poor prognosis in very young children with LQTS.[2,11] In the modern era, the use of pacemakers in these patients has been associated with an improved prognosis.[18] It is thought that this is achieved by reducing pause-dependent ventricular arrhythmias by limiting the repolarization dispersion seen during bradycardia.[48]

Effective pacing in very young children can be accomplished relatively easily using epicardial leads and abdominal generator placement. Although initial epicardial systems were prone to early lead failure, newer steroid-eluding leads function on par with endocardial leads.[49] As the morbidity for epicardial pacemaker system placement is relatively low, and there is potential to provide an effective means of rhythm stabilization, pacemaker placement should be considered for any very young patient with LQTS with AVB.

It should be noted, however, that patients with severe symptoms or recurrent syncope may not respond as well to pacemaker placement, even with beta-blockers.[50] In these patients, additional therapies may be needed, such as left cardiac sympathetic denervation or implantation of a back-up ICD.

Left Cardiac Sympathetic Denervation

Left cardiac sympathetic denervation has been advocated for the treatment of high-risk patients with LQTS.[51] In the largest study of this technique involving 147 patients, Schwartz and colleagues[51] showed a significant reduction in subsequent cardiac events for patients with LQTS who underwent denervation. Not all patients benefited, however, and Schwartz and colleagues[51] recommended that the procedure be reserved for patients with recurrent syncope despite beta-blockade and in patients who experience arrhythmia storms with an ICD.

Because of concerns regarding the development of Horner syndrome and other complications, as well as concerns regarding the reproducibility of results, the technique has not seen widespread use in the pediatric population. Collura, however, demonstrated that denervation could be successfully achieved from a video-assisted approach without complications in small children.[52] Among the 11 patients who underwent video-assisted thoracic surgery for secondary prevention of ventricular arrhythmias in this study, 5 were patients with LQTS who were younger than 1 year. All of the patients, including the 5 very young patients, had a marked reduction in cardiac events after surgery and none were felt to have any complications related to the surgery itself.

Considering the poor prognosis of very young children who present with severe symptoms, this technique should be considered as an adjunct to therapy and a center with experience performing this procedure in children should be sought.

ICD

There are limited data regarding the use of ICDs in very young children with LQTS. Although there are no data specific to very small children, ICD use in children is discussed. ICDs are effective for preventing SCD in children, including those with LQTS[53–55]; however, their use in the pediatric population is associated with a high rate of inappropriate shocks and system failure.[53,55] The use of ICDs in very young children presents the additional problem of the need for novel approaches to implantation because the small size of these children imposes limitations to vascular access.[56]

Benefits

In a study focused on LQTS in children, Etheridge and colleagues[55] reported that 5 of 19 of these children received an appropriate shock with a mean time to first shock of 18 ± 22 months from implantation. In separate larger studies by Berul and colleagues[53] and Heersche and colleagues[54] involving a more broad population of children receiving ICDs for various indications, the rate of appropriate discharges in children with primary electrical heart disease was approximately 23% to 37% and did not differ from that seen in children who underwent ICD implantation with different diagnoses. Not surprisingly, the rate of appropriate discharge was higher in patients who underwent ICD implantation for secondary prevention rather than primary prevention in this mixed diagnostic group.[53] Importantly, the time to first appropriate shock often occurred years after implantation.[53,54] Also important is the observation that ICDs may not be effective in all children with LQTS. Heersche and colleagues[54] reported that of 15 children with LQTS who received an ICD, 2 children died owing to refractory ventricular arrhythmias and electrical storm.

Risks

Although ICDs can save the lives of children at risk, their use is associated with significant morbidity. The rate of inappropriate shocks for pediatric patients was similar in Berul and colleagues'[53] study (24%) and Heersche and colleagues'[54] study (27%). Berul and colleagues[53] showed that children who underwent ICD for primary electrical disorders were more likely to receive an inappropriate shock than those who underwent ICD with cardiomyopathy (31% vs 13%, $P<.001$).[53] In addition to a high rate of inappropriate shocks, children suffer from a high rate of system failures and require frequent reintervention. Etheridge and colleagues[55] reported that nearly half of the pediatric patients with LQTS who underwent ICD or pacemaker insertion required device-related reintervention. Therefore, the overall morbidity of ICD implantation in children is high and must be taken into account when recommending an ICD for any child.

Novel Approaches

Although it may be technically feasible to place an endocardial system in some larger infants, this approach is highly discouraged. This approach is associated with a rate of vascular occlusion, which is directly related to the child's size.[57] For this reason, the traditional method for placing an ICD in a very young child involves placement of epicardial patches for defibrillation in conjunction with an epicardial pace-sense lead. These systems have gone out of favor because of the potential for fibrosis and calcification of the patches, which leads to restrictive physiology in some patients

and makes replacement of the patches extremely difficult.

To avoid the complications related to endocardial lead placement or epicardial patches, several innovatiove ICD configurations have been tried in very young children, as well as in other children with specific types of congenital heart disease that prohibit endocardial access.[47,56] These systems generally include placement of the generator in the abdomen. Defibrillation has been provided by several different configurations, in isolation or in conjunction with one another including the following:

- Subcutaneous arrays
- Subcutaneous patches
- Placement of an endocardial defibrillation lead in the pericardium and attached to the base of the heart.

An epicardial pace-sense lead is also placed to provide adequate arrhythmia detection and back pacing if necessary (**Fig. 5**). These systems have been shown to provide adequate energy for

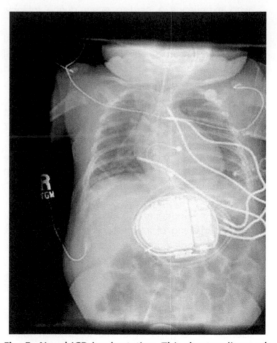

Fig. 5. Novel ICD implantation. This chest radiograph demonstrates a patient with LQTS with a novel ICD configuration consisting of an epicardial pace-sense lead, subcutaneous array around the left hemithorax, and an abdominal generator pocket location. (*From* Stephenson EA, Batra AS, Knilans TK, et al. A multicenter experience with novel implantable cardioverter defibrillator configurations in the pediatric and congenital heart disease population. J Cardiovasc Electrophysiol 2006;17:41–6; with permission.)

defibrillation[56]; however, as the child grows and the amount of energy required to defibrillate increases proportionally to the child's mass, the original configuration may need to be supplemented with additional arrays, patches, or leads. In addition to this, the original configuration may fail with slippage of these arrays, patches, and leads, which results in them being out of position as these children grow.[56] Movement of the endocardial leads placed in the pericardium has also been associated with cardiac strangulation as the lead tightens around the base of the heart. Although these novel systems can provide life-saving protection, they should be reserved for very small children with highly symptomatic LQTS and should be closely monitored as the child grows.

REFERENCES

1. Schwartz PJ, Stramba-Badiale M, Crotti L, et al. Prevalence of the congenital long-QT syndrome. Circulation 2009;120:1761–7.
2. Spazzolini DV, Mullally BS, Moss AJ, et al. Clinical implications for patients with long QT syndrome who experience a cardiac event during infancy. J Am Coll Cardiol 2009;54:832–7.
3. Horigome H, Nagashima M, Sumitomo N, et al. Clinical characteristics and genetic background of congenital long-QT syndrome diagnosed in fetal, neonatal, and infantile life: a national questionnaire survey in Japan. Circ Arrhythm Electrophysiol 2010;3:10–7.
4. Garson A, Dick M, Fournier A, et al. The long Qt syndrome in children: an international study of 287 patients. Circulation 1993;87:1866–72.
5. Arnestad M, Croti L, Rognum TO, et al. Prevalence of long-QT syndrome gene variants in sudden infant death syndrome. Circulation 2007;115:361–7.
6. Chang RK, Rodriguez S, Gurvitz M. Electrocardiogram screening of infants for long QT syndrome: survey of pediatric cardiologists in North America. J Electrocardiol 2010;43:4–7.
7. Priori SG, Napolitano C, Schwartz PJ. Low penetrance in the long-QT syndrome: clinical impact. Circulation 1999;99:529–33.
8. Petko C, Bradley DJ, Tristani-Firouzi M, et al. Congenital long QT syndrome in children identified by family screening. Am J Cardiol 2008;101:1756–8.
9. Hendricks KS, Grosfeld FJ, van Tintelen JP, et al. Can parents adjust to the idea that their child is at risk for a sudden death? Psychological impact of risk for long QT syndrome. Am J Med Genet A 2005;138A:107–12.
10. Lupoglazoff JM, Denjoy I, Villain E, et al. Long QT syndrome in neonates: conduction disorders associated with HERG mutations and sinus bradycardia with KCNQ1 mutations. J Am Coll Cardiol 2004;43:826–30.
11. Trippel DL, Parsons MK, Gillette PC. Infants with long-QT syndrome and 2:1 atrioventricular block. Am Heart J 1995;130:1130–4.
12. Zareba W, Moss AJ, Schwartz PJ, et al. Influence of the genotype on the clinical course of the long-QT syndrome. N Engl J Med 1998;339:960–5.
13. Moss AJ, Zareba W, Hall J, et al. Effectiveness and limitations of b-blocker therapy in congenital long-QT syndrome. Circulation 2000;101:616–23.
14. Hobbs JB, Peterson DR, Moss AJ, et al. Risk of aborted cardiac arrest or sudden cardiac death during adolescence in the long-QT syndrome. JAMA 2006;296:1249–54.
15. Goldenberg I, Moss AJ, Peterson DR, et al. Risk factors for aborted cardiac arrest and sudden cardiac death in children wit the congenital long-Qt syndrome. Circulation 2008;117:2184–91.
16. Hofbeck M, Ulmer H, Beinder E, et al. Prenatal findings in patients with prolonged QT interval in the neonatal period. Heart 1997;77:198–204.
17. Vincent GM. The heart rate of Romano-Ward syndrome patients. Am Heart J 1986;112:61–4.
18. Aziz PF, Tanel RE, Zelster IJ, et al. Congenital long QT syndrome and 2:1 atrioventricular block: an optimistic outcome in the current era. Heart Rhythm 2010;7:781–5.
19. Priori SG, Schwartz PJ, Napolitano C, et al. Risk stratification in the long-QT syndrome. N Engl J Med 2003;348:1866–74.
20. Krous HF, Beckwith JB, Byand RW, et al. Sudden infant death syndrome and unclassified sudden infant deaths: a definitional and diagnostic approach. Pediatrics 2004;114:234.
21. Minino AM, Heron MP, Smith BL. Deaths: preliminary data for 2004. Natl Vital Stat Rep 2006;54:31.
22. AAP Task Force on SIDS. The changing concept of sudden infant death syndrome: diagnostic coding shifts, controversies regarding the sleeping environment, and new variables to consider in reducing risk. Pediatrics 2003;116:1245.
23. Schwartz PJ. Cardiac sympathetic innervation and the sudden infant death syndrome: a possible pathologic link. Am J Med 1976;60:167–72.
24. Schwartz PJ, Stramba-Badiale M, Segantini A, et al. Prolongation of the QT interval and the sudden infant death syndrome. N Engl J Med 1998;338:1709–14.
25. Walsh SZ. Electrocardiographic intervals during the first week of life. Am Heart J 1963;66:36–41.
26. Van Norstrand DW, Ackerman MJ. Sudden infant death syndrome: do ion channels play a role? Heart Rhythm 2009;6:272–8.
27. Schwartz PJ, Priori SG, Bloise R, et al. Molecular diagnosis in a child with sudden infant death syndrome. Lancet 2001;358:1342–3.

28. Ackerman MJ, Siu BL, Sturner WQ, et al. Postmortem molecular analysis of SCN5A defects in sudden infant death syndrome. JAMA 2001;286:2264–9.

29. Marijon E, Tafflet M, Celermajer DS, et al. Sports-related sudden death in the general population. Circulation 2011;124:672–81.

30. Schwartz PJ, Moss AJ, Vincent GM, et al. Diagnostic criteria for the long QT syndrome. An update. Circulation 1993;88:782.

31. Hofman N, Wilde AA, Kaab S, et al. Diagnostic criteria for congenital long QT syndrome in the era of molecular genetics: do we need a scoring system? Eur Heart J 2007;28:575.

32. Fujimoto Y, Matsumoto T, Honda N, et al. Prenatal diagnosis of long QT syndrome by non-invasive fetal electrocardiography. J Obstet Gynaecol Res 2009; 35:555–61.

33. Moss AJ, Zareba W, Benhorin J, et al. ECG T-wave patterns in genetically distinct forms of the hereditary long QT syndrome. Circulation 1995;92:2929–32.

34. Funck-Brentano C, Jaillon P. Rate-corrected QT interval: techniques and limitations. Am J Cardiol 1993;72:17B.

35. Gow RM, Ewald B, Lai L, et al. The measurement of the QT and QTc on the neonatal and infant electrocardiogram: a comprehensive reliability assessment. Ann Noninvasive Electrocardiol 2009;14:165–75.

36. Goldenberg I, Mathew J, Moss AJ, et al. Corrected QT variability in serial electrocardiograms in long QT syndrome. J Am Coll Cardiol 2006;48:1047–52.

37. Quaglini S, Rognoni C, Priori SG, et al. Cost-effectiveness of neonatal ECG screening for the long QT syndrome. Eur Heart J 2006;27:1824–32.

38. Van Hare GF, Perry J, Berul CI, et al. Letters to the Editor: cost-effectiveness of neonatal ECG screening for the long QT syndrome. Eur Heart J 2007;28:137–41.

39. Maron BJ, Thompson PD, Ackerman MJ, et al. Recommendations and considerations related to pre-participation screening for cardiovascular abnormalities in competitive athletics: 2007 update: a scientific statement from the American Council on Nutrition, Physical Activity, and Metabolism: endorsed by the American College of Cardiology Foundation. Circulation 2007;115:1643–55.

40. Tester DJ, Will ML, Haglund CM, et al. Effect of clinical phenotype on yield of long QT syndrome genetic testing. J Am Coll Cardiol 2006;47:764–8.

41. Schwartz PJ, Garson A, Paul T, et al. Guidelines for the interpretation of the neonatal electrocardiogram. Eur Heart J 2002;23:1329–44.

42. Priori SG, Napolitano C, Schwartz PJ, et al. Association of long QT syndrome loci and cardiac events among patients treated with B-blockers. JAMA 2004;292:1341–4.

43. Liu JF, Jons C, Moss AJ, et al. Risk factors for recurrent syncope and subsequent fatal or near-fatal events in children and adolescents with long QT syndrome. J Am Coll Cardiol 2011;57:941–50.

44. Kaufman ES, McNitt S, Moss AJ, et al. Risk of death in the long QT syndrome when a sibling has died. Heart Rhythm 2008;5:831–6.

45. Moss AJ, Windle JR, Jall WJ, et al. Safety and efficacy of flecainide in subjects with long QT-3 syndrome (DeltaKPQ mutation): a randomized, double-blind, placebo controlled clinical trial. Ann Noninvasive Electrocardiol 2005;10:59–66.

46. Ten Harkel AD, Witsenburg M, d Jong PL, et al. Efficacy of an implantable cardioverter defibrillator in a neonate with LQT3 associated arrhythmias. Europace 2005;7:77–84.

47. Cuneo BF, Ovadia M, Strasburger JF, et al. Prenatal diagnosis and in utero treatment of torsades de pointes associated with congenital long QT syndrome. Am J Cardiol 2003;91:1395–8.

48. Shimizu W, Antzelevitch C. Differential effects of beta-adrenergic agonists and antagonists in LQT1, LQT2 and LQT3 models of the long QT syndrome. J Am Coll Cardiol 2000;35(3):778.

49. Cohen MI, Bush DM, Vetter VL, et al. Permanent epicardial pacing in pediatric patients: seventeen years of experience and 1200 outpatient visits. Circulation 2001;103:2585–90.

50. Dorostkar PC, Eldar M, Belhassen B, et al. Long term follow-up of patients with long-QT syndrome treated with beta-blockers and continuous pacing. Circulation 1999;100(24):2431.

51. Schwartz PJ, Priori SG, Cerrone M, et al. Left cardiac sympathetic denervation in the management of high-risk patients affected by the long-QT syndrome. Circulation 2004;109:1826–33.

52. Collura CA, Johnson JN, Moir C, et al. Left cardiac sympathetic denervation for the treatment of long QT syndrome and catecholaminergic polymorphic ventricular tachycardia using video-assisted thoracic surgery. Hear Rhythm 2009;6:752–9.

53. Berul CI, Van Hare GF, Kertesz NJ, et al. Results of a multicenter retrospective implantable cardioverter-defibrillator registry of pediatric and congenital heart disease patients. J Am Coll Cardiol 2008;51:1685–91.

54. Heersche JH, Blom NA, Van De Heuvel F, et al. Implantable cardioverter defibrillator therapy for prevention of sudden cardiac death in children in the Netherlands. Pacing Clin Electrophysiol 2010;33:179–85.

55. Etheridge SP, Sanatani S, Cohen MI, et al. Long QT Syndrome in the era of implantable defibrillators. J Am Coll Cardiol 2007;50:1335–40.

56. Stephenson EA, Batra AS, Knilans TK, et al. A multicenter experience with novel implantable cardioverter defibrillator configurations in the pediatric and congenital heart disease population. J Cardiovasc Electrophysiol 2006;17:41–6.

57. Figa FH, McCrindle BW, Bigras JL, et al. Risk factors for venous obstruction in children with transvenous pacing leads. Pacing Clin Electrophysiol 1997;20(8 Pt 1):1902–9.

The Role of the Sympathetic Nervous System in the Long QT Syndrome: The Long Road from Pathophysiology to Therapy

Peter J. Schwartz, MD, FESC[a,b,c,d,e,*]

KEYWORDS

- Long QT syndrome • Sympathetic imbalance
- Left cardiac sympathetic denervation
- Arrhythmic sudden death

The topic to be reviewed here is not neutral to me. Indeed, it has shaped much of my adult life. Accordingly, this article is written in a more personal style than is usually expected in a scientific article. It is to be hoped that the science will not be distorted by the waves of personal memories. As the role of the sympathetic nervous system in the long QT syndrome (LQTS) is tightly linked to my professional development and life, I have reviewed it as part of a narration that aims at being scientifically sound and, at the same time, interesting for the reader who is comfortable with a nontraditional approach.

HOW IT STARTED

In December 1970, in the days of black-and-white TV in Italy, an 18-year-old girl died suddenly during a live show watched by most Italians. The anchorman asked her a question, all cameras turned on her, she jumped up, and died. The girl had lost consciousness several times before whenever she became emotional. No diagnosis had been made. Later, I found an electrocardiogram (ECG) of the girl, made after a fainting episode. It showed a major prolongation of the QT interval that had gone completely unnoticed. The mother of the dead girl, and of the girl's 10 siblings, realized that a younger sister of her dead daughter had the same symptoms: sudden loss of consciousness, especially during emotional stress. The mother insisted on having the 9-year-old admitted to a leading hospital. She was admitted to the Department of Medicine of University Hospital in Milan, and specifically to 1 of the 4 beds for which I, a rookie barely out of medical school, had responsibility while beginning to learn practical medicine and cardiology.

The only obvious things were a very long QT interval (**Fig. 1**A) and the history of frequent syncope, always associated with physical or emotional stress. It really looked like a case of the sympathetic nervous system acting as a killer. No one had any idea of what disease the little

[a] Department of Molecular Medicine, University of Pavia, c/o Fondazione IRCCS Policlinico S. Matteo, V.le Golgi 19, 27100 Pavia, Italy
[b] Department of Cardiology, Fondazione IRCCS Policlinico S. Matteo, V.le Golgi 19, 27100 Pavia, Italy
[c] Cardiovascular Genetics Laboratory, Department of Medicine, Hatter Institute for Cardiovascular Research in Africa, The Cape Heart Centre, University of Cape Town Medical School Campus, Cape Town, South Africa 8001
[d] Department of Medicine, University of Stellenbosch, PO Box 19063, Tygerberg 7505, Cape Town, South Africa
[e] Department of Family and Community Medicine, College of Medicine, King Saud University, PO Box 2925, Riyadh 11461, Kingdom of Saudi Arabia
* Department of Molecular Medicine, University of Pavia, c/o Fondazione IRCCS Policlinico S. Matteo, V.le Golgi 19, 27100 Pavia, Italy.
E-mail address: peter.schwartz@unipv.it

Card Electrophysiol Clin 4 (2012) 75–85
doi:10.1016/j.ccep.2012.01.002
1877-9182/12/$ – see front matter © 2012 Elsevier Inc. All rights reserved.

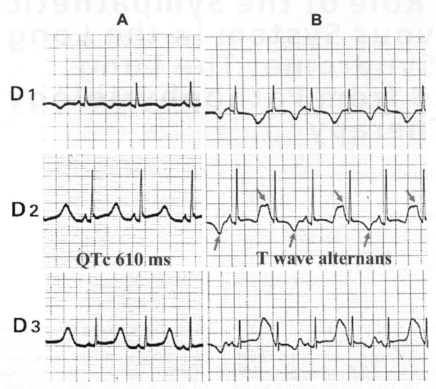

Fig. 1. (*A*) Control condition, QTc 610 milliseconds. (*B*) During fright. Tracings in (*B*) are simultaneous. Alternation of the T wave, in amplitude (D1) and in polarity (D2 and D3), is evident (*see arrows*). (*From* Schwartz PJ, Malliani A. Electrical alternation of the T wave. Clinical and experimental evidence of its relationship with the sympathetic nervous system and with the long QT syndrome. Am Heart J 1975;89:46; with permission.)

girl, named Agostina, had. Eventually a pediatric cardiologist recalled having seen something connecting QT prolongation and sudden death in the young; it had appeared in *The Lancet*, but he did not remember when. It was actually an editorial reporting on a case of familial sudden death in children published in Ireland,[1,2] which stimulated a hasty letter by an Italian pediatrician who wanted the world to know that 1 year earlier he had actually published a strikingly similar case in Italy.[3,4] When the cases were referred to as the Romano-Ward syndrome, everyone was happy. However, this helped me only a little because we still had no idea what we were really dealing with or how to treat Agostina. Given that her syncopal episodes were clearly triggered by sympathetic activation, we decided to initiate therapy with propranolol. Meanwhile, I began to read anything that might have linked QT-interval prolongation and sudden death.

While Agostina was in hospital, we brought her to the exercise stress test room, but she was frightened by the instrumentation and almost fainted: the ECG immediately recorded showed bizarre T-wave changes, which prompted one of the senior cardiologists to utter "ugly T waves."

I had no idea what was going on, but was quick enough to make a long recording of the episode. After looking at these strange T waves (**Fig. 1**B), which none of my seniors had been able to explain, I returned to the library. It did not take too long to learn that the phenomenon was called T-wave alternans, and was both rare and of uncertain significance. It took me a little time to review all of the few publications (30–40 patients worldwide) dealing with LQTS in its 2 variants, the Romano-Ward and the Jervell and Lange-Nielsen syndromes,[5] and to discover, with great excitement, that in half of them episodes of T-wave alternans had been noted. A rare phenomenon in an extremely rare disease? Very unlikely. There must have been a connection, and I was going to look for it.

Meanwhile, β-blocker therapy markedly reduced Agostina's syncopal episodes, but in the summer of 1972 she had a frank cardiac arrest and was resuscitated by her mother, who performed thump-version following our instructions. It was obvious that β-blockers were not enough for her.

My literature search proved useful because it led to the critical 1966 study by Frank Yanowitz, a student working with Abbie Abildskov, who showed in dogs that the QT interval was prolonged by right stellectomy and by left stellate stimulation, and shortened by left stellectomy.[6] This study called attention to the relation between cardiac sympathetic nerves and ventricular repolarization, and also prompted the first left cardiac sympathetic denervation (LCSD) performed by Moss and McDonald in 1971 in an LQTS patient not protected by β-blockers.[7] Before proceeding with actual nerve section, Moss and McDonald performed transient pharmacologic blockade of the 2 stellate ganglia and reported that block of the right was followed by appearance of T-wave alternans. My simple reasoning was that if the link existed between the 2 phenomena, it should have been possible to elicit T-wave alternans by the same sympathetic manipulation that was prolonging the QT interval. As Agostina's episodes of syncope were occurring during sympathetic activation, I focused on electrical stimulation of the left stellate ganglion. Such a focus was possible for me because, although working in a department of medicine, my group was mostly involved in basic physiology focused on single-fiber recording from the cardiac sympathetic nerves.[8] After several unsuccessful experiments, I eventually succeeded in reproducing in anesthetized cats both QT prolongation and striking episodes of T-wave alternans (**Fig. 2**).[9] This finding is what led me to think, and shortly afterward to propose more formally, that LQTS was related to some sort of imbalance in the sympathetic innervation of the heart with left-sided dominance. The sympathetic imbalance hypothesis was born. Almost.

In the meantime I had to take care of Agostina. Having become convinced that neural activity through the left stellate ganglion was playing an important detrimental role, I somehow convinced her parents, and on March 25, 1973, Agostina underwent LCSD by removal of the lower half of

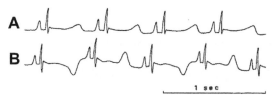

Fig. 2. Anesthetized cat: ECG (D2). (*A*) Control; (*B*) 5 seconds after the cessation of a 30-second electrical stimulation of both stellate ganglia (left ganglion: 20 V, 2 milliseconds, 20 Hz; right ganglion: 10 V, 2 milliseconds, 20 Hz). Alternation in polarity of the T wave is evident. (*From* Schwartz PJ, Malliani A. Electrical alternation of the T wave. Clinical and experimental evidence of its relationship with the sympathetic nervous system and with the long QT syndrome. Am Heart J 1975;89:47; with permission.)

the left stellate ganglion and of the first 4 thoracic ganglia. It is gratifying to be able to say that in the almost 40 subsequent years she had no more cardiac events, that I served as best man at her wedding, and that she comes to see me for her regular visit every year. By chance, our lives crossed at the right time and we affected each other's future in a unique way: I probably saved her life and she, by stimulating me to study the intriguing disease that was affecting her, shifted my professional life and career in an unforeseen direction, with long-lasting consequences that I do not regret.

ONE HYPOTHESIS AND MANY EXPERIMENTS

My first question was "what type of imbalance?" Indeed, it could have been dependent either on a higher-than-normal left or on a lower-than-normal right cardiac sympathetic activity. I knew, from the experiments by Randall and Rohse[10] in 1964, that the sympathetic control of heart rate was largely dependent on the right stellate ganglion, meaning that a lower-than-normal right cardiac sympathetic activity had to be accompanied by a lower-than-normal heart rate, something that was easy to verify. Sure enough, most of the existing clinical reports were mentioning surprisingly low resting heart rates in the LQTS children. It was then that I was ready to propose that LQTS was caused by a sympathetic imbalance secondary to, more often than not, a reduced right sympathetic activity. This was done in 1975.[11]

What was lost in the subsequent literature was that this concept was always presented as a still unproved working hypothesis. Moreover, the training in basic physiology taught me prudence in writing, and despite my young age I was very cautious with written words. It is good science to read the original publications carefully. As early as 1975, just after having presented the hypothesis, I added "...however, the possibility cannot be ruled out that some local myocardial abnormality might also be involved in the pathogenesis of the disease. In such a case, the sympathetic stimulations would only trigger the syncopal episodes."[11] Ten years later, while more fully proposing sympathetic imbalance based on new experimental data (see below), I was even more cautious as I wrote the following:

The particularly high arrhythmogenic potential of the left-sided nerves leaves open the possibility that the basic defect in LQTS is an unknown intracardiac abnormality that decreases electrical stability and makes the myocardium more vulnerable to the effect of sympathetic discharges. In this case the sympathetic nervous system, acting mostly through the quantitatively dominant left stellate ganglion, would merely represent the trigger for ventricular tachyarrhythmias.[12]

Twenty-five years later it is evident that what I was referring to as the "unknown intracardiac abnormality" has revealed itself for the genetic abnormalities that have transformed the entire field, and specifically LQTS. By simply replacing the "unknown intracardiac abnormality" with "genetic mutations," I can still stand by what I wrote so long ago.

However, the hypothesis as proposed in 1975 was not really explaining the relationship between sympathetic imbalance and arrhythmogenesis. Accordingly, in the subsequent years I tried to address this intriguing issue and focused on what seemed the key issues: "does a reduced right cardiac sympathetic activity really increase arrhythmia risk?" and "does removal of the left cardiac sympathetic nerves really prevent life-threatening arrhythmias?" In the next paragraphs I will succinctly review the main experimental findings.

In anesthetized dogs, by circulating a coolant around either the right or the left stellate ganglion, we were able to produce a transient unilateral block. By rewarming the ganglia we were able to go back to control conditions and repeat the procedure several times during the same experiment. As a stimulus we used a brief (maximum 90 seconds) occlusion of a coronary artery, which was performed either in control conditions or during blockade of one of the stellate ganglions. The main finding, totally unexpected by that time (and which prompted one reviewer to bluntly dismiss it because "this must be an artifact") was that ischemia-induced arrhythmias were increased by right stellate ganglion block and were markedly decreased by left stellate ganglion block (**Fig. 3**).[13]

The LQTS patients, however, do not have ischemia-related arrhythmias; they have a high propensity to develop ventricular fibrillation. Therefore, I turned to ventricular fibrillation threshold (VFT), a reliable quantitative marker of cardiac electrical instability, which is inversely related to the probability that a single premature beat will induce ventricular fibrillation. Our finding was that VFT was lowered by right stellate ganglion block and markedly increased by left stellate ganglion block (**Fig. 4**).[14] Right and left sympathectomy provided the same results. The implications were not minuscule. If patients affected by LQTS really had a lower-than-normal right cardiac sympathetic activity, the findings were explaining why they were

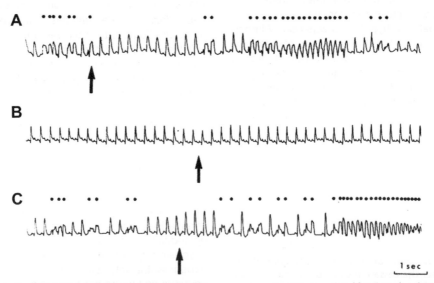

Fig. 3. Effect of a 90-second occlusion of the circumflex coronary artery in an animal having the descending coronary artery ligated at the beginning of the experiment, in control conditions, and during left stellate ganglion blockade (SGB). (*A*) Coronary artery occlusion (CAO) in control conditions. Episodes of ventricular tachycardia (VT) before and after release (*see arrows*) of the occlusion with several premature ventricular contractions (PVCs). (*B*) CAO during left SGB. No arrhythmias. (*C*) CAO in control conditions. There are several PVCs followed by VT, which a few seconds later precipitates in ventricular fibrillation. (*A*), (*B*), and (*C*) are consecutive trials. The black dots indicate ectopic beats. (*From* Schwartz PJ, Stone HL, Brown AM. Effects of unilateral stellate ganglion blockade on the arrhythmias associated with coronary occlusion. Am Heart J 1976;92:595; with permission.)

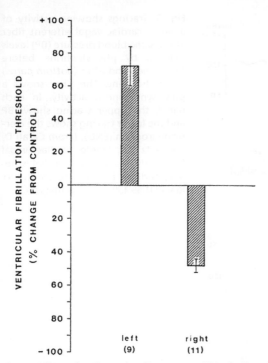

Fig. 4. Effect of unilateral stellectomy and blockade on the ventricular fibrillation threshold. Left stellectomy or blockade (9 animals) raised the ventricular fibrillation threshold by 72% ± 12% compared with control values (P<.001). Right stellectomy or blockade (11 animals) lowered the ventricular fibrillation threshold by 48% ± 3% (mean ± SE) compared with control values. (*Modified from* Schwartz PJ, Snebold NG, Brown AM. Effects of unilateral cardiac sympathetic denervation on the ventricular fibrillation threshold. Am J Cardiol 1976;37:1036; with permission.)

so easily catapulted into ventricular fibrillation by sympathetic activation. On the other hand, our results were also providing a very strong rationale for removing the left stellate ganglion because following this intervention, independently of possible changes in the QT interval, it would have been much more difficult to develop ventricular fibrillation. These data, however, had implications clearly beyond LQTS. Indeed, they strongly suggested that adequate LCSD, which in man means removal of the lower half of the left stellate ganglion together with the first 3 to 4 thoracic ganglia (see Appendix),[15] could reduce the propensity toward ventricular fibrillation, certainly in those clinical conditions in which life-threatening arrhythmias are triggered by sympathetic activation, but possibly also in other settings.

These 2 studies[13,14] clearly strengthened the sympathetic imbalance hypothesis, but were also fully consistent with the possibility that the role of the sympathetic nervous system was primarily that of a trigger.[11,12] Come what may, there were important implications for therapy and I set out to explore them.

The rationale for LCSD has been discussed several times, and the interested reader can find adequate information not only in the original articles but also, more broadly or more succinctly, in 2 reviews[16,17] written across an interval of 25 years. Accordingly, here I merely summarize the main findings. LCSD was found to not affect cardiac performance during exercise,[18] to slightly increase heart rate during exercise,[18] and to not produce postdenervation supersensitivity.[19] Relevant to ischemic heart disease is that LCSD increases myocardial reactive hyperemia, which means that it increases the ability of the coronary bed to dilate,[20] and potentially relevant to heart failure[21,22] is that LCSD leads to an increase in reflex vagal activity (**Fig. 5**).[23]

A clear and undeniable merit of the "sympathetic imbalance" hypothesis is that, independently of its validity and in order to either dismiss it or confirm it, it has stimulated a large number of studies that have provided meaningful and novel information with implications for the management of LQTS and other diseases.

DISCOVERIES AND REFLECTIONS: A MOMENT OF PAUSE

A large clap of thunder was heard on March 31, 1995, and lightning struck. The identification of the first 2 genes for LQTS,[24,25] followed a few months later by the identification of the third,[26] was much more than a revolution. It had a major impact on cardiology and turned upside-down the understanding of LQTS. Out goes the sympathetic imbalance hypothesis, in come the genes. A moment of pause was required, and some reflections.

Put very simply, the following could and can be said: (1) LQTS is caused by mutations on a growing number of genes, 13 at the last count[27]; (2) LQTS in not caused by a sympathetic imbalance; (3) what was proposed in 1975 and in 1985 was eminently correct when it was indicated that the causative mechanism might have been a still "unknown intracardiac abnormality," which in 1995 was found to be a genetic abnormality; and (4) the role of the sympathetic nervous system as a trigger remained entirely intact, with clear implications for therapy. Accordingly, the rest of this article is devoted to discussing the role of cardiac sympathetic denervation in the management of life-threatening disorders, with special reference to LQTS.

While still pausing to reflect, I find it tempting to express an unlikely but nevertheless intriguing

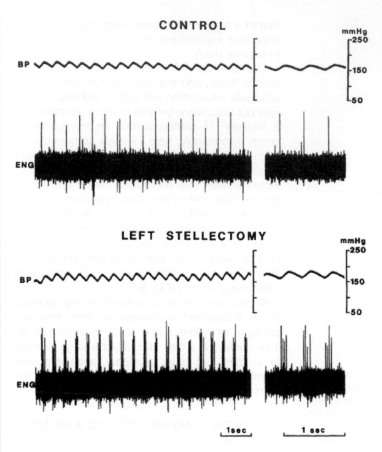

CONTROL

LEFT STELLECTOMY

Fig. 5. Tracings showing activity of a single cardiac vagal efferent fiber at the same blood pressure (BP) levels induced by phenylephrine before (*top panel*) and after (*bottom panel*) left stellectomy. The fiber shows a pulse-synchronous activity. In each panel, the upper tracing shows BP and the lower tracing shows the electroneurogram (ENG). (*From* Cerati D, Schwartz PJ. Single cardiac vagal fiber activity, acute myocardial ischemia, and risk for sudden death. Circ Res 1991;69:1398; with permission.)

possibility, which requires a step back. When in 1976 I proposed that some of the victims of sudden infant death syndrome (SIDS) might have died because of a mechanism the same or similar to that of LQTS,[28] a hypothesis fully confirmed more than 30 years later,[29] I indicated that one possibility was that of a sympathetic imbalance simply reflecting the biological reality that most physiologic parameters are normally distributed, according to the Gaussian curve. This possibility implies that some infants are born at the extremes of the curve and specifically that some will have either a low right-sided or a high left-sided cardiac sympathetic activity; namely, a condition that is associated with a prolonged QT interval[6] and with an increased susceptibility to life-threatening cardiac arrhythmias.[13,14] This seems an unavoidable reality. Could it apply to LQTS? Probably not, but in the absence of any supporting data and just for the sake of the argument, I would say that, in theory, a fraction of the 15-20% of patients certainly affected by LQTS, who are genotype negative, and who are the only affected members in their families, might by chance be at

the extremes of the normal distribution for cardiac sympathetic innervation and might behave almost exactly as typical genetically mediated LQTS patients. Yes, I know I will never be able to prove this; however, it will also be impossible to disprove it.

THE ROLE OF LEFT CARDIAC SYMPATHETIC DENERVATION IN THE PREVENTION OF SUDDEN DEATH

As I have already discussed the rationale for LCSD, I now focus on its therapeutic effects, dealing first with LQTS and then with other conditions.

LCSD for LQTS

In 1975 I reported on the first successful experience in 3 patients not protected by β-blockers.[12] By 1991 this number had increased to 85 patients,[30] and in 2004 I and my colleagues published a large collaborative report on 147 patients.[31] We are currently in the process of revisiting the worldwide data but the 2004 report is discussed here. The patients were considered at very high risk for 3 reasons: they were almost all (99%) symptomatic and 47% had survived a cardiac arrest, 75% of them had recurrent cardiac events despite full-dose β-blockade, and their average QTc was extraordinarily prolonged (543 ± 65 milliseconds). Given the current use of an implantable cardioverter-defibrillator (ICD) in anyone with an aborted cardiac arrest, the interest is primarily on those patients without cardiac arrest. Over a mean follow-up of 8 years, mortality in this high-risk group was 3%. It is interesting that QTc shortened by an average of 40 milliseconds, a biologically relevant change. Of additional relevance, also for other medical conditions, are the data on 5 patients with electrical storms and multiple shocks. These unfortunate youngsters had a mean of 29 shocks per person per year in the 2 years following ICD implant; in the 4 years following LCSD this number decreased to 3 shocks per person per year, reflecting the complete suppression in 4 and some persistence in 1. This reduction by 95% in LQTS patients with electrical storms had an obvious and dramatic effect on the quality of life of these patients and their families.

Cardiologists are responsible for providing their patients with a full disclosure of the treatment options available regardless of their personal views on the approach to follow for preventing life-threatening arrhythmias, to which they are of course entitled and which they are expected to share with their patients. When dealing with patients at risk for arrhythmic death, it should no longer be acceptable to deny at-risk patients their right to complete information about the advantages and disadvantages of LCSD. Failure to do so may carry medicolegal implications.[32]

For too many years most of these interventions have been performed at my institution, or by our surgeon with whom I have been traveling to several countries (China, the Netherlands, Russia, Israel, and others) to teach local surgeons. The technique used has been described in detail (see Appendix).[15] An important recent development has been that both the Boston Children Hospital and the Mayo Clinic have begun to perform LCSD by thoracoscopy,[33,34] and are now using this approach frequently and successfully for high-risk patients.

We perform LCSD whenever a patient cannot be treated with β-blockers (eg, because of asthma), has breakthrough cardiac events on β-blocker therapy, has a daytime resting heart rate close to 40 beats per minute, or is regarded on medical grounds to remain at high risk despite medical therapy. We use LCSD for LQTS patients whenever they have had multiple ICD shocks.

LCSD for Other Medical Conditions

The most important disease for which we now often use LCSD is catecholaminergic polymorphic ventricular tachycardia (CPVT). In 2008 we provided the first report of its long-term efficacy in 3 such patients who had multiple episodes of ventricular tachycardia/ventricular fibrillation (VT/VF) with frequent ICD shocks,[35] and this was soon followed by similar reports.[33,34] We are in the process of reviewing the worldwide experience, and the current data on almost 20 patients are extremely encouraging. The rationale for LCSD is very strong. On the one hand, the arrhythmias in CPVT are triggered by increases in sympathetic activity, whether due to physical or emotional stress[36–38]; on the other hand, ICD implants in these patients are often the beginning of a nightmare because a life-saving shock, which generates pain and fear, very often initiates a deadly cycle of arrhythmias and shocks. Indeed, there is a growing number of reports on CPVT patients dying after multiple ICD shocks, not infrequently triggered by fast supraventricular arrhythmias.[39,40] For patients not fully protected by β-blockers, we recommend performing LCSD as a first step and, if necessary, the combination of an ICD (as a safety net to protect the patient's life) and LCSD to prevent as much as possible the initiation of a life-threatening arrhythmia and thus to preserve the quality of life of these patients. At present, this is what we are doing until the potential long-term benefit of flecainide is better established.[41]

In 1992 we provided evidence that LCSD could dramatically reduce the 1-year incidence of sudden cardiac death among high-risk patients after a myocardial infarction.[42] The patients had suffered an acute anterior wall myocardial infarction complicated by VT/VF in the first 24 hours. Patients were randomized to placebo, the β-blocker oxprenolol, and LCSD. The 1-year mortality in the placebo group was very high, 21.3%, and was strikingly reduced to 3.6% and 2.7%, respectively, by LCSD and oxprenolol. This study has also demonstrated the powerful antifibrillatory effect of LCSD in ischemic heart disease.

There are other diseases, such as hypertrophic cardiomyopathy and arrhythmogenic right ventricular cardiomyopathy, that are associated with a relatively high risk of sudden cardiac death, especially in specific subgroups. LCSD has not been used in these diseases, largely because at first glance the therapeutic rationale may not be immediately evident. However, the powerful antifibrillatory effect of LCSD[14] may very well be useful for some of these patients, especially in developing countries where the availability of ICDs for primary prevention is very limited, if not absent. This option is worthy of consideration when medical therapy is likely to be insufficient.

FINAL CONSIDERATIONS

It is interesting to revisit after 40 years the concepts related to a specific disease, in this case LQTS, and to see how they have evolved. Sympathetic imbalance, as originally proposed, is unlikely to contribute to the pathogenesis of LQTS but certainly plays a major role in triggering its life-threatening arrhythmias, as correctly proposed in 1975[11] and 1985.[12] The studies stimulated by the sympathetic imbalance hypothesis have generated many unsuspected novel data and have provided an extremely strong rationale for the therapeutic use of LCSD to prevent ventricular fibrillation, not only in LQTS but also in other life-threatening diseases associated with high risk for arrhythmic sudden death.

The lesson to be taken is, in my opinion, that scientific hypotheses can prove very useful even when they are entirely or partially incorrect, provided that sound and careful studies are performed with the goal to either confirm them or dismiss them while keeping an open mind for whatever the final result will be. It is in this way that science moves forward. The pleasure of traveling is not in reaching the destination but in walking along the road.

ACKNOWLEDGMENTS

The author is grateful to Pinuccia De Tomasi for expert editorial support. The Appendix of this article is reproduced from Odero A, Bozzani A, De Ferrari GM, et al. Left cardiac sympathetic denervation for the prevention of life-threatening arrhythmias. The surgical supraclavicular approach to cervico-thoracic sympathectomy. Heart Rhythm 2010;7:1161–5; with permission.

APPENDIX

LCSD: The Method Used in Pavia

The technique described here is the one we have been using since 1973. The average duration of the surgical intervention is 35 to 40 minutes. The patient is positioned supine on the operating table, with a roll beneath the shoulders, hyperextending the neck and turning the head to the right. Under single-lumen tracheal intubation general anesthesia, the supraclavicular approach is used. A small (5–6 cm) transverse incision is made 1 finger-breadth above the left clavicle, and the platysma and the clavicular head of the sternocleidomastoid muscle are transected (**Fig. 6**).

The internal jugular vein is identified just below the muscle, mobilized, and retracted medially. Care must be taken to avoid injury to the thoracic duct. The descending cervical lymphatic vessels join the thoracic duct at the junction of the subclavian vein and left internal jugular vein. The thoracic duct courses from posterior to anterior behind the jugular and subclavian veins to enter the superior border of the junction of these latter 2 vessels. Should injury to the thoracic duct occur, the duct must be identified and ligated to avoid a lymph fistula. The scalene fat pad is retracted laterally, and the anterior scalene muscle is identified lateral to the carotid artery. The phrenic nerve courses on

A   **B**

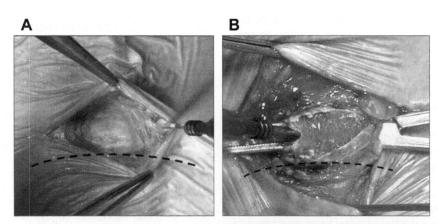

Fig. 6. Usual position for surgical incision. First the platysma (*A*) and then the clavicular head of the sternocleidomastoid muscle (*B*) are transected. Dotted line shows the course of underlying left clavicle. (*From* Odero A, Bozzani A, De Ferrari GM, et al. Left cardiac sympathetic denervation for the prevention of life-threatening arrhythmias. The surgical supraclavicular approach to cervico-thoracic sympathectomy. Heart Rhythm 2010; 7:1162; with permission.)

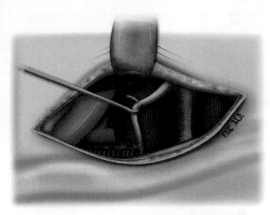

Fig. 7. The next surgical step, which consists of the identification and cautious mobilization of the phrenic nerve and the transection of the anterior scalene muscle. (*From* Odero A, Bozzani A, De Ferrari GM, et al. Left cardiac sympathetic denervation for the prevention of life-threatening arrhythmias. The surgical supraclavicular approach to cervico-thoracic sympathectomy. Heart Rhythm 2010;7:1163; with permission.)

the anterior surface of the scalene muscle, and must be identified and gently mobilized (**Fig. 7**).

Subsequently, the anterior scalene muscle is transected by cutting through a nonvascular area in the lower neck near its origin from the first rib. After the scalene muscle is transected, the subclavian artery is visible. It is retracted upward to obtain sufficient exposure of the thoracic ganglia. The subclavian vein lies under the clavicle and is not usually in the operative field. Behind the subclavian artery, the seventh cervical transverse

process is exposed along with the pleural dome. The apical pleura is freed from its ligament (Sibson fascia) and the lung is reflected caudally (**Fig. 8**).

It is usually possible to push the pleural dome downward and free it from its ligament through a digital dissection. The stellate ganglion and the second thoracic ganglion are thus easily exposed. The stellate lies in front of the Chassaignac tuberosity. This landmark helps to correctly identify the position of the stellate ganglion. When the stellate ganglion has been freed from its bed, the chain can often be followed down as far as the fourth thoracic ganglion. Care must be taken to avoid injury of the intercostals vessels. After local application of 1% lidocaine (**Fig. 9**), which is used to prevent injury currents that would produce a significant release of norepinephrine at ventricular level, the stellate ganglion is dissected in 2 halves, thus separating the first thoracic ganglion from the inferior cervical one, and the cephalic portion of the left stellate ganglion is preserved, to prevent Horner syndrome. The left cervicothoracic sympathectomy performed with this technique, which we refer to as left cardiac sympathetic denervation, involves removal of the lower half of the left stellate ganglion, together with thoracic ganglia T2 to T4 and its associated rami communicantes. This intervention provides adequate cardiac denervation with no or minimal Horner syndrome because most of the sympathetic fibers directed to the ocular region usually cross the upper portion of the left stellate ganglion and thus are spared. Because LCSD is performed by an extrapleural approach, thoracotomy and thoracic drainage are unnecessary. The dissected material is sent to the pathology

A

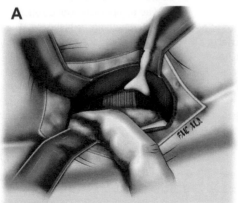

B

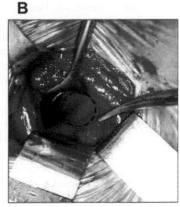

Fig. 8. The apical pleura is freed from its ligament, the lung is reflected caudally, and the subclavian artery is retracted upward. (*A*) Schematic diagram. (*B*) Intraoperative image. Black dashed circle shows underlying stellate ganglion. (*From* Odero A, Bozzani A, De Ferrari GM, et al. Left cardiac sympathetic denervation for the prevention of life-threatening arrhythmias. The surgical supraclavicular approach to cervico-thoracic sympathectomy. Heart Rhythm 2010;7:1163; with permission.)

A

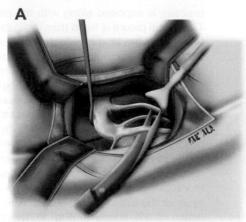

B

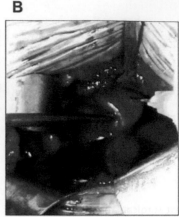

Fig. 9. Stellate ganglion and sympathetic chain are exposed (*A*, schematic drawing), and 1% lidocaine is injected (*B*, intraoperative image) before excision of the nerve to prevent injury currents and release of norepinephrine. (*From* Odero A, Bozzani A, De Ferrari GM, et al. Left cardiac sympathetic denervation for the prevention of life-threatening arrhythmias. The surgical supraclavicular approach to cervico-thoracic sympathectomy. Heart Rhythm 2010;7:1164; with permission.)

laboratory and read by frozen sections to ensure that nerve and ganglia have been removed.

REFERENCES

1. Congenital cardiac arrhythmia [editorial]. Lancet 1964; 284:26–7.
2. Ward OC. A new familial cardiac syndrome in children. J Ir Med Assoc 1964;54:103–6.
3. Romano C. Congenital cardiac arrhythmia. Lancet 1965;285:658–9.
4. Romano C, Gemme G, Pongiglione R. Aritmie cardiache rare dell'età pediatrica. Clin Pediatr 1963;45: 656–83.
5. Jervell A, Lange-Nielsen F. Congenital deaf-mutism, functional heart disease with prolongation of the Q-T interval, and sudden death. Am Heart J 1957; 54:59–68.
6. Yanowitz F, Preston JB, Abildskov JA. Functional distribution of right and left stellate innervation to the ventricles: production of neurogenic electrocardiographic changes by unilateral alteration of sympathetic tone. Circ Res 1966;18:416–28.
7. Moss AJ, McDonald J. Unilateral cervicothoracic sympathetic ganglionectomy for the treatment of long QT interval syndrome. N Engl J Med 1971; 285:903–4.
8. Malliani A, Schwartz PJ, Zanchetti A. A sympathetic reflex elicited by experimental coronary occlusion. Am J Physiol 1969;217:703–9.
9. Schwartz PJ, Malliani A. Electrical alternation of the T wave. Clinical and experimental evidence of its relationship with the sympathetic nervous system and with the long QT syndrome. Am Heart J 1975; 89:45–50.

10. Randall WC, Rohse WG. The augmentor action of the sympathetic cardiac nerves. Circ Res 1956;4: 470–5.
11. Schwartz PJ, Periti M, Malliani A. The long Q-T syndrome. Am Heart J 1975;89:378–90.
12. Schwartz PJ. Idiopathic long QT syndrome: progress and questions. Am Heart J 1985;109:399–411.
13. Schwartz PJ, Stone HL, Brown AM. Effects of unilateral stellate ganglion blockade on the arrhythmias associated with coronary occlusion. Am Heart J 1976;92:589–99.
14. Schwartz PJ, Snebold NG, Brown AM. Effects of unilateral cardiac sympathetic denervation on the ventricular fibrillation threshold. Am J Cardiol 1976; 37:1034–40.
15. Odero A, Bozzani A, De Ferrari GM, et al. Left cardiac sympathetic denervation for the prevention of life-threatening arrhythmias. The surgical supraclavicular approach to cervico-thoracic sympathectomy. Heart Rhythm 2010;7:1161–5.
16. Schwartz PJ. The rationale and the role of left stellectomy for the prevention of malignant arrhythmias. Ann N Y Acad Sci 1984;427:199–221.
17. Schwartz PJ. Cutting nerves and saving lives. Heart Rhythm 2009;6:760–3.
18. Schwartz PJ, Stone HL. Effects of unilateral stellectomy upon cardiac performance during exercise in dogs. Circ Res 1979;44:637–45.
19. Schwartz PJ, Stone HL. Left stellectomy and denervation supersensitivity in conscious dogs. Am J Cardiol 1982;49:1185–90.
20. Schwartz PJ, Stone HL. Tonic influence of the sympathetic nervous system on myocardial reactive hyperemia and on coronary blood flow distribution. Circ Res 1977;41:51–8.

21. Schwartz PJ, De Ferrari GM, Sanzo A, et al. Long term vagal stimulation in patients with advanced heart failure: first experience in man. Eur J Heart Fail 2008;10:884–91.

22. De Ferrari GM, Crijns HJ, Borggrefe M, et al, for the CardioFit Multicenter Trial Investigators. Chronic vagus nerve stimulation: a new and promising therapeutic approach for chronic heart failure. Eur Heart J 2011;32:847–55.

23. Cerati D, Schwartz PJ. Single cardiac vagal fibers activity, acute myocardial ischemia, and risk for sudden death. Circ Res 1991;69:1389–401.

24. Wang Q, Shen J, Splawski I, et al. SCN5A mutations associated with an inherited cardiac arrhythmia, long QT syndrome. Cell 1995;80:805–11.

25. Curran ME, Splawski I, Timothy KW, et al. A molecular basis for cardiac arrhythmia: HERG mutations cause long QT syndrome. Cell 1995;80:795–803.

26. Wang Q, Curran ME, Splawski I, et al. Positional cloning of a novel potassium channel gene: KvLQT1 mutations cause cardiac arrhythmias. Nat Genet 1996;12:17–23.

27. Schwartz PJ, Crotti L, Insolia R. Long QT syndrome: from genetics to management. Circ Arrhythm Electrophysiol, in press.

28. Schwartz PJ. Cardiac sympathetic innervation and the sudden infant death syndrome. A possible pathogenetic link. Am J Med 1976;60:167–72.

29. Arnestad M, Crotti L, Rognum TO, et al. Prevalence of long QT syndrome gene variants in sudden infant death syndrome. Circulation 2007;115:361–7.

30. Schwartz PJ, Locati EH, Moss AJ, et al. Left cardiac sympathetic denervation in the therapy of congenital long QT syndrome: a worldwide report. Circulation 1991;84:503–11.

31. Schwartz PJ, Priori SG, Cerrone M, et al. Left cardiac sympathetic denervation in the management of high-risk patients affected by the long QT syndrome. Circulation 2004;109:1826–33.

32. Schwartz PJ. Efficacy of left cardiac sympathetic denervation has an unforeseen side effect: medicolegal complications. Heart Rhythm 2010;7:1330–2.

33. Atallah J, Fynn-Thompson F, Cecchin F, et al. Video-assisted thoracoscopic cardiac denervation: a poten-tial novel therapeutic option for children with intractable ventricular arrhythmias. Ann Thorac Surg 2008;86:1620–5.

34. Collura CA, Johnson JN, Moir C, et al. Left cardiac sympathetic denervation for the treatment of long QT syndrome and catecholaminergic polymorphic ventricular tachycardia using video-assisted thoracic surgery. Heart Rhythm 2009;6:752–9.

35. Wilde AA, Bhuiyan ZA, Crotti L, et al. Left cardiac sympathetic denervation for catecholaminergic polymorphic ventricular tachycardia. N Engl J Med 2008;358:2024–9.

36. Leenhardt A, Lucet V, Denjoy I, et al. Catecholaminergic polymorphic ventricular tachycardia in children. A 7-year follow-up of 21 patients. Circulation 1995;91:1512–9.

37. Priori SG, Napolitano C, Memmi M, et al. Clinical and molecular characterization of patients with catecholaminergic polymorphic ventricular tachycardia. Circulation 2006;114:1012–9.

38. Hayashi M, Denjoy I, Extramiana F, et al. Incidence and risk factors of arrhythmic events in catecholaminergic polymorphic ventricular tachycardia. Circulation 2009;119:2426–34.

39. Mohamed U, Napolitano C, Priori SG. Molecular and electrophysiological bases of catecholaminergic polymorphic ventricular tachycardia. J Cardiovasc Electrophysiol 2007;18:791–7.

40. Pizzale S, Gollob MH, Gow R, et al. Sudden death in a young man with catecholaminergic polymorphic ventricular tachycardia and paroxysmal atrial fibrillation. J Cardiovasc Electrophysiol 2008;19:1319–21.

41. van der Werf C, Kannankeril PJ, Sacher F, et al. Flecainide therapy reduces exercise-induced ventricular arrhythmias in patients with catecholaminergic polymorphic ventricular tachycardia. J Am Coll Cardiol 2011;57:2244–54.

42. Schwartz PJ, Motolese M, Pollavini G, et al, the Italian Sudden Death Prevention Group. Prevention of sudden cardiac death after a first myocardial infarction by pharmacologic or surgical antiadrenergic interventions. J Cardiovasc Electrophysiol 1992;3:2–16.

The Role of the Implantable Cardioverter-Defibrillator in the Long QT Syndrome

Wojciech Zareba, MD, PhD*, Ilan Goldenberg, MD,
Arthur J. Moss, MD

KEYWORDS

- Implantable cardioverter defibrillator • Long QT syndrome
- Arrhythmia

The long QT syndrome (LQTS) is an inherited arrhythmia disorder manifested by corrected QT interval (QTc) prolongation in the electrocardiogram and a propensity to torsade de pointes ventricular tachycardia (VT), which might lead to sudden cardiac death (SCD), usually in young, otherwise healthy individuals.[1–4] It is estimated that LQTS is present in 1:2500 to 1:5000 in the general population. In about 70% to 75% of genotyped patients, specific gene abnormality can be identified.[5] To date, there are 13 genes with several hundred mutations identified in patients with LQTS.[5–7] The LQT1 and LQT2 types of LQTS account for about 45% each, and LQT3 accounts for about 5% to 8%, whereas the remaining types of LQTS are extremely rare.[4,7]

Management of patients with LQTS is intended to decrease the risk of cardiac events and sudden death.[6] The risk of cardiac events could be diminished by proper lifestyle changes: decreased risk of arousal and stress situations triggering cardiac events (alarm clocks, phone rings, exercise, water nbsp;activities), avoiding competitive sports, and avoidance of drugs known to prolong the QT interval. β-Blocker therapy, with its antiadrenergic effect (but also several other effects including sodium channel blocking effects), is the treatment of choice in patients with LQTS.[8–10] Some patients

benefit from antiadrenergic therapy consisting of left sympathetic cardiac denervation, further decreasing the probability of catecholaminergic triggers of arrhythmias.[11] QT shortening and stability of repolarization are goals of gene-specific pharmacologic therapies, but currently this approach is applied only to patients with LQT3 who seem to benefit from sodium channel blocker therapy.[12–14] The implantable cardiac defibrillator (ICD) is an important therapeutic option for patients with LQTS offering life-saving shocks and protection in patients who are at increased risk of developing VT/ventricular fibrillation.[15–17] Data regarding effects of different therapies, including ICD therapy, in patients with LQTS are based on nonrandomized observational studies, but growing and combined experience of several investigative groups provides the basis for the current therapeutic approach to management of patients with LQTS.

IDENTIFICATION OF HIGH-RISK PATIENTS WITH LQTS

In the last decade, physicians have been diagnosing significantly more patients with LQTS, including a wide spectrum of clinical presentations. Because ICD therapy is invasive and carries some risks, only high-risk patients with LQTS should be

Heart Research Follow-up Program, Cardiology Division, University of Rochester Medical Center, 265 Crittenden Boulevard, CU 420653, Rochester, NY 14642, USA
* Corresponding author.
E-mail address: wojciech_zareba@urmc.rochester.edu

Card Electrophysiol Clin 4 (2012) 87–95
doi:10.1016/j.ccep.2011.12.004

considered for such therapy. However, identification of high-risk patients with LQTS remains a challenge, and frequently ICDs are implanted based on physician and patient preference rather than using an evidence-based approach.

The clinical course of LQTS is influenced by many factors including QTc duration, history of syncope or cardiac arrest, age, gender, and genotype.[1–3,18–24]

The QTc interval duration is the primary electrocardiogram finding and serves as an important risk factor in patients with LQTS. Data from several studies documented that the risk of cardiac events is directly related to the length of the QTc interval.[1–3] In particular, QTc greater than 500 or greater than 550 milliseconds (**Fig. 1**) is associated with twofold to fourfold higher risk of aborted cardiac arrest (ACA) or death than is observed in patients with QTc less than 500 milliseconds.[21]

Prior history of syncopal episodes serves as an important risk factor. **Table 1**[21–25] and **Fig. 2** show data from the analysis of more than 1000 patients with LQTS with syncope.[25] The lowest risk was found in patients with only 1 syncopal episode occurring before the start of β-blocker therapy, whereas patients experiencing syncope after starting β-blocker therapy had a 3.6-fold increase in the risk of severe arrhythmic events relative to this low-risk group and displayed a risk of severe arrhythmic events similar to that of patients not treated with β-blockers.

Age and gender influence the risk of cardiac events (syncope, ACA, or death) in patients with LQTS.[18–25] Boys have a higher risk of cardiac events than girls during childhood, whereas after puberty this risk levels off, and girls show a steady increase after midadolescence.[18–24]

Table 1 Cox model for risk factors related to severe cardiac events in patients presenting with the first syncope event and repeated syncope events on and off β-blocker therapy			
Parameter	HR	95% CI	P Value
Syncopal episodes and β-blocker therapy	—	—	—
≥1 syncopal event on β-blocker therapy[a]	3.59	2.25–5.74	<.001
>1 Syncopal event off β-blocker therapy[a]	1.96	1.37–2.82	<.001
QTc interval >500 ms	1.76	1.32–2.27	<.001
Female subjects age 14–40 y[b]	1.86	1.40–2.49	<.001
Time-dependent β-blocker therapy	0.46	0.32–0.65	<.001

Abbreviations: CI, confidence interval; HR, hazard ratio.
[a] Relative to subjects with only 1 syncopal episode occurring while off β-blocker therapy.
[b] Relative to male subjects aged 14 to 40 years.
Data from Jons C, Moss AJ, Goldenberg I, et al. Risk of fatal arrhythmic events in LQTS patients after syncope. J Am Coll Cardiol 2010;55:783–8.

The risk of cardiac events varies by LQTS genotype, with patients with LQT1 and LQT2 (with mutations in genes encoding potassium channel proteins) having a higher risk of cardiac events than patients with LQT3 (caused by mutations in the sodium channel gene), but LQT3 is associated with increased lethality of cardiac events.[2–4] When analyzing ACA or death as an endpoint, patients with LQT3 have a higher risk of these events than

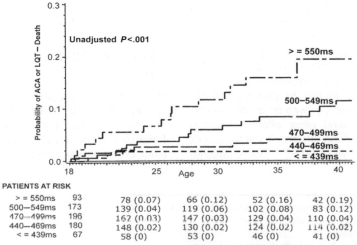

Fig. 1. QTc and the risk of aborted cardiac arrest (ACA) or SCD during adulthood. (*From* Sauer AJ, Moss AJ, McNitt S, et al. Long QT syndrome in adults. J Am Coll Cardiol 2007;49:332; with permission.)

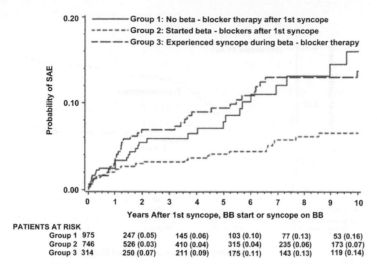

Fig. 2. The cumulative risk of ACA, ICD shock, and death (1) after first syncope off β-blocker therapy, (2) after start of β-blocker therapy, or (3) if syncope occurs during β-blocker therapy. (*From* Jons C, Moss AJ, Goldenberg I, et al. Risk of fatal arrhythmic events in LQTS patients after syncope. J Am Coll Cardiol 2010;55:785; with permission.)

patients with LQT1 and LQT2 in childhood until age 18 years and in adults after age 40 years, but there is no difference in the risk of these severe events at age 18 to 40 years.[4,21]

A combination of age, gender, QTc, history of syncope, and genotype should influence clinical decisions regarding preventive or therapeutic measures in patients with LQTS. **Table 2** shows comprehensive information regarding the risk of ACA or death by age categories using these clinical parameters.[4]

Because genotype is of limited use when evaluating the risk of ACA or death in patients with LQTS, risk-factor identification could be enriched with information regarding location of mutation, presence of multiple mutations, or nature of the ion channel kinetic abnormality.[26,27] In patients with LQT1 (**Fig. 3**, top), a transmembrane mutation location identifies a twofold increased risk for cardiac events compared with non–transmembrane mutation locations.[26] In patients with LQT2 (see **Fig. 3**, bottom), mutations in the transmembrane S5 to S6 loop location were associated with an increased risk of cardiac events.[27]

Schwartz and colleagues[17] developed a scoring system to identify patients with ICD at high risk for cardiac events (**Table 3**). The so-called M-FACT score is an acronym derived from M (−1 point for being free of cardiac events while on therapy for >10 years), F (QTc 500–550 milliseconds), A (age ≤20 or >20 years at implantation), C (cardiac arrest), and T (events on therapy). As shown in **Fig. 4**, patients with incremental values of the score had worse event-free survival.

Table 2
High-risk subsets for ACA or SCD by age groups[a]

Age Group	High-Risk Subsets
Childhood (1–12 y)	Men with prior syncope and/or QTc >500 ms Women with prior syncope
Adolescence (13–20 y)	Men and women with one or more of the following: • QTc ≥530 ms • ≥1 episode of syncope in the past 1 y • ≥2 episodes of syncope in the past 2–10 y
Adulthood (20–40 y)	One or more of the following: • Female gender • Interim syncope after age 18 y • QTc ≥500 ms
41–60 y[b]	One or more of the following: • Female gender • Syncope in the past 10 y • QTc ≥500 ms • LQT3 genotype
61–75 y[b]	Syncope in the past 10 y

[a] Findings are from separate multivariable Cox models in each age group for the end point of ACA or SCD.
[b] Because LQTS-related events are more difficult to delineate in the older age group, the end point in the age group of 41 to 60 years comprised ACA or death from any cause.
Data from Goldenberg I, Zareba W, Moss AJ. Long QT syndrome. Curr Probl Cardiol 2008;33:629–94.

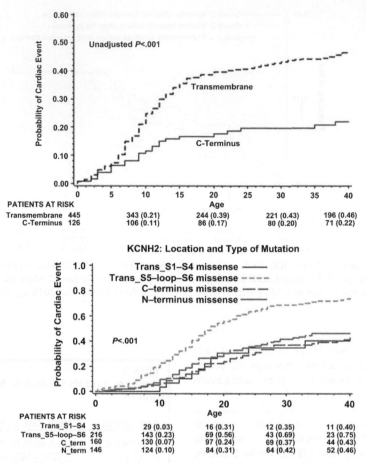

Fig. 3. Cumulative probability of cardiac events by mutation location in patients with LQT1 (*upper panel*) and LQT2 (*bottom panel*). (Upper panel: *From* Moss AJ, Shimizu W, Wilde AA, et al. Clinical aspects of type-1 long-QT syndrome by location, coding type, and biophysical function of mutations involving the KCNQ1 gene. Circulation 2007;115:2486; with permission; Lower panel: *From* Shimizu W, Moss AJ, Wilde AA, et al. Genotype-phenotype aspects of type 2 long QT syndrome. J Am Coll Cardiol 2009;54:2057; with permission.)

CLINICAL PROFILE AND OUTCOME OF PATIENTS WITH LQTS TREATED WITH ICDS

Clinical reports on ICD use in patients with LQTS have limited numbers of patients. Groh and colleagues[15] described the use of the ICD in 35 patients with LQTS, of whom approximately three-fourths had experienced prior ACA before implantation. During mean follow-up of 31 (± 21)

Table 3
The M-FACT[a] risk score for evaluating LQTS patient risk of appropriate ICD therapy

	−1 Point	0 Points	1 Point	2 Points
Event free on therapy for >10 years	Yes	—	—	—
QTc (ms)	—	≤500	>500–<550	>550
Prior ACA	—	No	Yes	—
Events on therapy	No	Yes	—	—
Age at implantation (y)	—	>20	≤20	—

[a] Acronym derived from M (−1 point for being free of cardiac events while on therapy for >10 years), F (QTc 500–550 ms), A (age≤20 or >20 years at implantation), C (cardiac arrest), and T (events on therapy).
Data from Schwartz PJ, Spazzolini C, Priori SG, et al. Who are the long-QTsyndrome patients who receive an implantable cardioverter-defibrillator and what happens to them? Data from the European long-QT syndrome implantable cardioverter-defibrillator (LQTS ICD) Registry. Circulation 2010;122:1272–82.

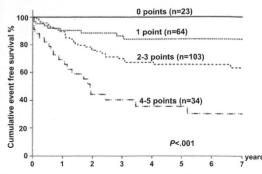

Fig. 4. Cumulative event-free survival for a first appropriate ICD shock according to an increasing M-FACT risk score. (*From* Schwartz PJ, Spazzolini C, Priori SG, et al. Who are the long-QT syndrome patients who receive an implantable cardioverter-defibrillator and what happens to them? data from the European long-QT syndrome implantable cardioverter-defibrillator (LQTS ICD) registry. Circulation 2010;122:1278; with permission.)

months, 21 experienced 1 or more appropriate ICD therapies and there were no deaths.

In 2003, we reported ICD experience in 125 patients with LQTS with ICDs from the Rochester LQTS ICD Registry,[16] of whom 54 (43%) had a history of ACA, 19 (15%) had syncope despite β-blocker treatment, 44 (35%) had history of syncope before therapy, and, in 8 (7%), sudden death in the family was the only contributing factor (apart from QTc prolongation). Mean age at implantation was 23 years and mean QTc was 517 milliseconds. **Fig. 5** shows a 16% cumulative risk of appropriate ICD therapy at 4 years in these patients, translating into a risk of about 4% per year. Subsequent analysis of 100 patients with genotype data showed (**Fig. 6**) that the highest risk of ventricular arrhythmias requiring ICD shocks was observed in patients with 2 LQTS-related mutations and with LQT2 mutations.[28]

This study also compared the clinical course of 125 LQTS ICD recipients with 161 matched

patients with LQTS who met similar clinical criteria for ICD implantation but were managed medically without an ICD because of patient or physician preference. In the 73 high-risk ICD-treated patients, 1 death (1.3%) occurred during an average follow-up of 3 years, whereas, in the non-ICD patients, 26 deaths (16%) occurred during a follow-up of 8 years.

In 2010, Schwartz and colleagues[17] reported data from the European registry on 233 patients with LQTS with ICD. Similarly to the US cohort, mean QTc was 516 milliseconds, mean age at implantation of 30 years was higher than 23 years in the US cohort, 44% had a history of ACA (similar to 43% in the US cohort), and 47% had syncope (similar to 50% in the US cohort). During a average 4.6-year follow-up, appropriate ICD therapy was received by 28% of patients (**Fig. 7**), with a 4-year risk estimated from the figure at about 30%. Seven patients died, including 6 of noncardiac causes and 1 of a nonarrhythmic cardiovascular event. Despite similarities in mean QTc and proportion of patients with ACA and syncope, European patients with ICDs showed a higher risk of arrhythmic events requiring appropriate ICD therapy than US patients with ICDs. This finding could be attributed to different genetic profiles of the studied patients, or possibly differences in ICD programming. Analysis of 141 genotyped patients in the European cohort also showed the highest risk of events in patients with double mutations, but, unlike the US cohort, patients with LQT1 had a higher risk of events than patients with LQT2 and LQT3 (**Fig. 8**). However, data from both studies are from retrospective registries and do not represent cohorts with prespecified criteria for ICD indications.

CURRENT GUIDELINES FOR ICD INDICATIONS IN LQTS

The American College of Cardiology/American Heart Association/Heart Rhythm Society *2008 Guidelines for Device-Based Therapy of Cardiac Rhythm Abnormalities*[29] established recommendations for ICD that are relevant for patients with LQTS. The guidelines include indication classes categorized as follows:

- Class I: procedure/treatment should be performed/administered
- Class IIa: it is reasonable to perform/administer procedure/treatment
- Class IIb: procedure/treatment may be considered
- Class III: procedure/treatment should not be performed/administered

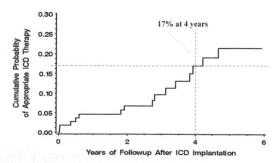

Fig. 5. Cumulative probability of ICD therapy in 125 patients with LQTS enrolled in the US LQTS ICD Registry.

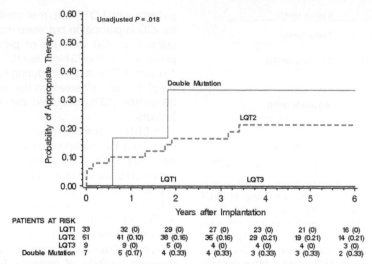

Fig. 6. Risk of appropriate therapy by genotype in 100 patients in the US LQTS ICD Registry. (*From* Zareba W, Goldenberg I, Moss AJ, et al. Implantable cardioverter-defibrillator therapy by genotype in long QT syndrome patients. Heart Rhythm 2007;4(Suppl):S131; with permission.)

At the same time, information is provided regarding evidence substantiation given indications categorized as follows:

- Level A: multiple populations were evaluated and the data were derived from multiple randomized clinical trials or registries in a large number of individuals
- Level B: limited populations evaluated and the data derived from a single randomized trial or nonrandomized studies
- Level C: very limited populations and the consensus was based on the opinions of experts, case series, or standard of care

Using these principles of classification of treatment indications, the following recommendations for ICD are applicable to patients with LQTS:

Class I

ICD therapy is indicated in patients who are survivors of cardiac arrest caused by ventricular fibrillation or hemodynamically unstable sustained VT after evaluation to define the cause of the event and to exclude any completely reversible causes (*level of evidence: A*).

This indication is a general one for secondary prevention of sudden death caused by cardiac

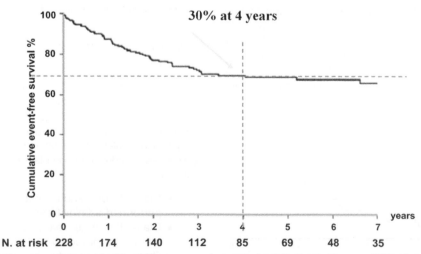

Fig. 7. Cumulative event-free survival for a first appropriate ICD shock in the European LQTS ICD Registry. (*From* Schwartz PJ, Spazzolini C, Priori SG, et al. Who are the long-QT syndrome patients who receive an implantable cardioverter-defibrillator and what happens to them? data from the European long-QT syndrome implantable cardioverter-defibrillator (LQTS ICD) Registry. Circulation 2010;122:1276; with permission.)

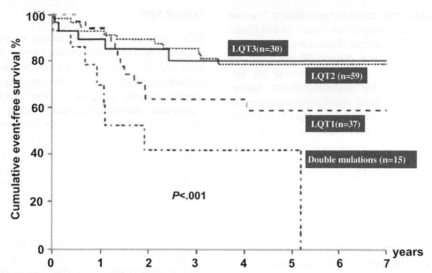

Fig. 8. Risk of appropriate therapy by genotype in 144 European ICD registry patients by genotype. (*From* Schwartz PJ, Spazzolini C, Priori SG, et al. Who are the long-QT syndrome patients who receive an implantable cardioverter-defibrillator and what happens to them? data from the European long-QT syndrome implantable cardioverter-defibrillator (LQTS ICD) Registry. Circulation 2010;122:1278; with permission.)

arrest and it also applies to patients with LQTS. Level of evidence A attributed to this indication is derived from the studies evaluating the role of ICDs in cardiac arrest survivors among patients with postinfarction and nonischemic cardiomyopathy. There is no level A evidence for supporting ICD implantation after cardiac arrest in patients with LQTS. Evidence at level B could be considered for this agreed-on indication.

Class IIa

ICD implantation is reasonable to reduce SCD in patients with LQTS who are experiencing syncope and/or VT while receiving β-blockers (level of evidence: B).

This indication is probably the most frequently exercised in patients with LQTS based on observational studies and clinical experience.

Class IIb

ICD therapy may be considered for patients with LQTS and risk factors for SCD (level of evidence: B).

There are data for factors identifying increased risks of sudden death or cardiac arrest in patients with LQTS (as described earlier), but there are limited data documenting the usefulness of ICDs in such patients.

The class I and IIa indications discussed earlier seem obvious and well justified with cardiac arrest, syncope, and/or documented VT despite β-blocker therapy. The biggest challenge concerns patients with syncope before β-blocker therapy. In such patients, syncope alone is probably insufficient to

qualify patients for ICD without exercising pharmacologic therapy first. The decision regarding ICD therapy in a young patient with the prospect of numerous generator replacements and possible complications during the next 40 to 50 years cannot be taken lightly. Therefore, in patients with a first syncopal episode without β-blockers, data from risk-stratification studies of patients with LQTS could be applied. As indicated in **Table 2**, a combination of clinical and genetic factors might identify high-risk individuals who might benefit from ICD even though they had a syncopal episode without β-blocker therapy, especially with QTc prolongation (>500 milliseconds). High-risk mutations associated with specific mutation locations might further assist in the decision (eg, transmembrane location of mutations in patients with LQT1, transmembrane S5–S6 loop location of mutation in patients with LQT2, or multiple LQTS-related mutations).[26,27] There is a tendency to elect ICD treatment in patients with LQT3 even without prior events,[16,17,28] based on data indicating higher lethality of cardiac events in patients with LQT3 than in patients with LQT1 and LQT2.[2] However, there are not enough data supporting such practices and physicians should take into account QTc prolongation and history of cardiac events as the primary reasons to consider ICDs in patients with LQT3.

COMPLICATIONS OF ICD THERAPY

Inappropriate ICD therapy represents a significant challenge in all patients with ICDs, including patients with LQTS. In these usually young individuals, abnormal sensing, specifically T-wave oversensing, is of particular concern. In the European study,[17] inappropriate shocks were observed in 25 patients (11%) and, among 86 documented inappropriate shocks, 51 were caused by abnormal sensing, 21 by supraventricular tachycardia, and 12 by lead fracture/dislodgement. Current devices have more robust algorithms minimizing the risk of inappropriate therapy caused by T-wave oversensing. Therefore, it is thought that this complication will occur less frequently with improved technology. There is no clear recommendation regarding optimal device programming to minimize the risk of inappropriate therapy caused by supraventricular tachyarrhythmias without compromising treatment of VT/ventricular fibrillation. Because episodes of torsade de pointes in patients with LQTS have a tendency to self-terminate, a long delay and a higher threshold VT zone might be needed. There is a need for further research regarding optimal programming of ICDs in patients with LQTS.

As with other conditions requiring ICD therapy, there are complications at the time of the implantation procedure as well as after implantation. The frequency of these complications is similar to that observed in patients with more common indications for ICDs. In the study by Schwartz and colleagues,[17] 15 of 233 patients (6%) experienced major adverse events including perforation, tamponade, lead revisions requiring open chest surgery, and device-related infection/endocarditis. In addition, 40 patients (17%) had minor adverse events. ICD therapy is associated with a significant number of major and minor adverse events and proper selection of patients is of primary importance.

ICD implantation in the pediatric population poses specific challenges. This topic is discussed in the article by Blaufox elsewhere in this issue.

COST-EFFECTIVENESS OF ICD IN PATIENTS WITH LQTS

In LQTS,[29] defibrillator therapy was shown to be cost-effective in high-risk male patients (incremental cost-effectiveness ratio [ICER] = $3328 per quality-adjusted life-year saved), and cost saving in high-risk women (ICER = $7102 gained per quality-adjusted life-year saved) and very high-risk men and women (ICER = $15,483 and $19,393 gained per quality-adjusted life-year saved, respectively). Defibrillator therapy was not shown to be cost-effective in low-risk patients with LQTS (ICER in the range of $400,000–$600,000 lost per quality-adjusted life-year saved). These data further indicate the need for proper patient selection.

SUMMARY

ICD implantation is a frequently exercised therapeutic option in management of high-risk patients with LQTS. Proper selection of usually young patients for this invasive therapy requires experienced clinical judgment. The evidence from numerous risk-stratification studies in patients with LQTS shows that the following factors should be considered as indicating high risk for ACA or death: QTc prolongation, history of ACA, history of syncope (especially on β-blockers), and information on location and type of mutations. A combination of these factors might be particularly useful when considering ICD in patients without classic indications (ie, those without cardiac arrest or without syncope on β-blocker therapy). Recent syncope off β-blocker therapy, QTc greater than 500 milliseconds, and the high-risk nature of LQTS mutations could be considered as a set of variables that indicate a high risk of life-threatening ventricular arrhythmias and may justify ICD implantation in patients with LQTS with such characteristics. Further studies are needed.

REFERENCES

1. Moss AJ, Schwartz PJ, Crampton RS, et al. The long QT syndrome. Prospective longitudinal study of 328 families. Circulation 1991;84:1136–44.
2. Zareba W, Moss AJ, Schwartz PJ, et al. Influence of genotype on the clinical course of the long-QT syndrome. International Long-QT Syndrome Registry Research Group. N Engl J Med 1998;339:960–5.
3. Priori SG, Schwartz PJ, Napolitano C, et al. Risk stratification in the long-QT syndrome. N Engl J Med 2003;348:1866–74.
4. Goldenberg I, Zareba W, Moss AJ. Long QT syndrome. Curr Probl Cardiol 2008;33:629–94.
5. Napolitano C, Priori SG, Schwartz PJ, et al. Genetic testing in the long QT syndrome. Development and validation of an efficient approach to genotyping in clinical practice. JAMA 2005;294:2975–80.
6. Zareba W, Cygankiewicz I. Long QT syndrome and short QT syndrome. Prog Cardiovasc Dis 2008;51:264–78.
7. Splawski I, Shen J, Timothy KW, et al. Spectrum of mutations in long-QT syndrome genes: KVLQT1, HERG, SCN5A, KCNE1, and KCNE2. Circulation 2000;102:1178–85.
8. Moss AJ, Zareba W, Hall WJ, et al. Effectiveness and limitations of beta-blocker therapy in congenital long-QT syndrome. Circulation 2000;101:616–23.
9. Priori SG, Napolitano C, Schwartz PJ, et al. Association of long QT syndrome loci and cardiac events among patients treated with β-blockers. JAMA 2004;292:1341–4.

10. Goldenberg I, Bradley J, Moss A, et al. Beta-blocker efficacy in high-risk patients with the congenital long-QT syndrome types 1 and 2: implications for patient management. J Cardiovasc Electrophysiol 2010;21:893–901.

11. Schwartz PJ, Priori SG, Cerrone M, et al. Left cardiac sympathetic denervation in the management of high-risk patients affected by the long-QT syndrome. Circulation 2004;109:1826–33.

12. Schwartz PJ, Priori SG, Locati EH, et al. Long QT syndrome patients with mutations on the SCN5A and HERG genes have differential responses to Na+ channel blockade and to increases in heart rate. Implications for gene-specific therapy. Circulation 1995;92:3381–6.

13. Windle R, Geletka RC, Moss AJ, et al. Normalization of ventricular repolarization with flecainide in long QT syndrome patients with SCN5A: DeltaKPQ mutation. Ann Noninvasive Electrocardiol 2001;6:153–8.

14. Moss AJ, Zareba W, Schwarz KQ, et al. Ranolazine shortens repolarization and improves myocardial relaxation in patients with type-3 long QT syndrome. J Cardiovasc Electrophysiol 2008;19:1289–93.

15. Groh WJ, Silka MJ, Oliver RP, et al. Use of implantable cardioverter-defibrillators in the congenital long QT syndrome. Am J Cardiol 1996;78:703–6.

16. Zareba W, Moss AJ, Daubert JP, et al. Implantable cardioverter defibrillator in high-risk long QT syndrome patients. J Cardiovasc Electrophysiol 2003;14:337–41.

17. Schwartz PJ, Spazzolini C, Priori SG, et al. Who are the long-QT syndrome patients who receive an implantable cardioverter-defibrillator and what happens to them? data from the European Long-QT Syndrome Implantable Cardioverter-Defibrillator (LQTS ICD) Registry. Circulation 2010;122:1272–82.

18. Zareba W, Moss AJ, le Cessie S, et al. Risk of cardiac events in family members of patients with long QT syndrome. J Am Coll Cardiol 1995;26:1685–91.

19. Zareba W, Moss AJ, Locati EH, et al. Modulating effects of age and gender on the clinical course of long QT syndrome by genotype. J Am Coll Cardiol 2003;42:103–9.

20. Locati EH, Zareba W, Moss AJ, et al. Age- and sex-related differences in clinical manifestations in patients with congenital long-QT syndrome: findings from the International LQTS Registry. Circulation 1998;97:2237–44.

21. Sauer AJ, Moss AJ, McNitt S, et al. Long QT syndrome in adults. J Am Coll Cardiol 2007;49:329–37.

22. Hobbs JB, Peterson DR, Moss AJ, et al. Risk of aborted cardiac arrest or sudden cardiac death during adolescence in the long-QT syndrome. JAMA 2006;296:1249–54.

23. Goldenberg I, Moss AJ, Peterson DL, et al. Risk of aborted cardiac arrest or sudden cardiac death in children with the congenital long-QT syndrome. Circulation 2008;117:2184–91.

24. Goldenberg I, Moss AJ, Bradley J, et al. Long QT after age 40. Circulation 2008;117:2192–201.

25. Jons C, Moss AJ, Goldenberg I, et al. Risk of fatal arrhythmic events in LQTS patients after syncope. J Am Coll Cardiol 2010;55:783–8.

26. Moss AJ, Shimizu W, Wilde AA, et al. Clinical aspects of type-1 long-QT syndrome by location, coding type, and biophysical function of mutations involving the KCNQ1 gene. Circulation 2007;115:2481–9.

27. Shimizu W, Moss AJ, Wilde AA, et al. Genotype-phenotype aspects of type 2 long QT syndrome. J Am Coll Cardiol 2009;54:2052–62.

28. Zareba W, Goldenberg I, Moss AJ, et al. Implantable cardioverter-defibrillator therapy by genotype in long QT syndrome patients. Heart Rhythm 2007; 4(Suppl):S131.

29. Goldenberg I, Moss AJ, Maron BJ, et al. Cost-effectiveness of implanted defibrillators in young people with inherited cardiac arrhythmias. Ann Noninvasive Electrocardiol 2005;10(Suppl 4):67–83.

How to Interpret Results of Genetic Testing and Counsel Families

Raffaella Bloise, MD[a,b], Silvia G. Priori, MD, PhD[a,b,c],*

KEYWORDS

- Genetic testing • Long QT syndrome
- Molecular diagnostics • Counseling

The successful completion of the human genome project has facilitated the identification of disease-causing genes and has promoted the introduction of DNA screening in clinical medicine. In turn, the application of molecular diagnostics to patient management has generated the need to design novel models of care for patients with inherited diseases.

Patients affected by life-threatening inherited arrhythmogenic disorders should be under the care of a team of clinicians with expertise in the diagnosis and management of these diseases to ensure that they have access to physicians able to provide accurate diagnosis, optimal therapy selection, and appropriate interpretation of the results of DNA analysis, including a comprehensive discussion on the pros and cons of extending genetic studies to family members.

At the present time, only a limited number of arrhythmia clinics can offer a specialized consultation for patients with long QT syndrome (LQTS) and any of the other channelopathies. The complex interpretation of genetic results, as well as the impact that genetic results may have on prognosis and response to therapy, call for the development of a specific educational track to train arrhythmologists in this new subspecialty of clinical electrophysiology.

This article discusses the complexity of the interpretation of genetic testing in LQTS with a specific focus on (1) who should be screened, (2) what to expect from the screening of LQTS genes, and (3) when and why genetic screening should be extended to family members. The challenges that are present in the interpretation of genetic results and the tools that may overcome the hurdle posed by unknown DNA variants are also discussed.

WHO SHOULD BE SCREENED FOR MUTATIONS IN LQTS GENES?

DNA analysis for the identification of mutations that cause mendelian diseases has become an important diagnostic tool for the management of families affected by inherited diseases. In the most straightforward situation, mutation screening is performed in the index case of a family affected by a mendelian disorder. In this setting, genetic screening is usually requested to allow the identification of a mutation that can be used to extend genetic evaluation to all family members so that only the mutation carriers are directed to clinical evaluation. However, genetic testing may also be requested in individuals in whom the diagnosis of a heritable disease is not firmly established and, therefore, DNA analysis becomes the last step of the diagnostic investigation.

When patients are evaluated because they present clinical profiles compatible with LQTS but not

[a] Molecular Cardiology, IRCCS Fondazione Salvatore Maugeri, Pavia, Italy
[b] Department of Molecular Medicine, University of Pavia, Pavia, Italy
[c] Cardiovascular Genetics Program, Leon H. Charney Division of Cardiology, NYU Langone Medical Center, New York, NY, USA
* Corresponding author. Cardiology Division and Molecular Cardiology, Salvatore Mageri Foundation 10/10A, Pavia 27100, Italy.
E-mail address: silvia.priori@fsm.it

Card Electrophysiol Clin 4 (2012) 97–101
doi:10.1016/j.ccep.2012.01.003
1877-9182/12/$ – see front matter

conclusively diagnostic for the disease, it is important to establish a detailed family history as well as a comprehensive clinical evaluation of at least first-degree family members before requesting genetic screening. If, despite the clinical evaluation of family members, the diagnosis of LQTS has not clearly emerged in the family, it is reasonable to complete the diagnostic evaluation with genetic screening of the index case.

WHAT TO EXPECT FROM THE SCREENING OF LQTS GENES

As discussed earlier, genetic testing in LQTS may be requested in patients with a confirmed clinical diagnosis and in individuals with a possible or with a probable diagnosis; the objective of requesting genetic testing in the 2 settings are different and they are discussed later.

When mutation screening in LQTS genes is requested in a proband with an uncertain diagnosis of LQTS, the primary goal of the requesting physician is to verify whether it is possible to establish a conclusive diagnosis of the disease through the identification of an LQTS-causing mutation. In this setting, whenever a pathogenetic mutation is identified, it becomes important to extend the genetic screening to family members of the index case to identify all the mutation carriers in the family. If genetic screening is not conclusive (ie, no mutation is identified), the diagnosis of LQTS remains uncertain given that a negative result does not exclude the diagnosis of LQTS because the patient may still carry a mutation in one of the LQTS genes that have not yet been identified. Another possible result of DNA screening is the identification of a DNA variant of unknown significance (VUS); in this setting, it is not possible to confirm or dismiss an LQTS diagnosis. When a VUS is identified in the index case, there is no value in screening for such a mutation in the family members.

When genetic screening is performed in a patient with a sound clinical diagnosis of LQTS, the test is usually requested because the genetic variant of LQTS in a given patient helps predict the probability of experiencing life-threatening arrhythmias, and it also helps in estimating the response to β-blocker therapy. The value of genetic screening for risk stratification is discussed elsewhere in this issue by Mazzanti and colleagues.

One important difference between performing genetic screening in probands with a conclusive diagnosis of LQTS versus screening individuals with a borderline QT interval is the much lower percentage of successfully genotyped individuals lacking a conclusive diagnosis of LQTS. We performed a cost analysis[1] for genetic screening in patients with LQTS and showed that, based on the identification of a disease-causing mutation in 64% of patients with a clinically robust diagnosis of LQTS, the cost per positively genotyped patient was approximately US $8418. In contrast, when screening was performed in individuals in whom LQTS diagnosis was only suspected based on borderline corrected QT interval (QTc), the percentage of positive genetic diagnosis was reduced to 14%, raising the cost per positive genotyped individual to US $37,565. These data call for a careful and appropriate use of genetic screening in patients with a reasonable suspicion of LQTS.

WHEN AND WHY GENETIC SCREENING SHOULD BE EXTENDED TO FAMILY MEMBERS

It is important to extend genetic screening to family members of an index case in whom a disease-causing mutation has been identified. This recommendation reflects the position of the "Heart Rhythm Society (HRS)/European Heart Rhythm Association (EHRA) Consensus Document on Genetic Screening in Channelopathies and Cardiomyopathies."[2] However, few considerations can be made because of the debated issue of the ethical and legal implications of molecular diagnosis of an inherited condition in asymptomatic individuals and in individuals devoid of clinical manifestations of the disease.

When extending genetic testing to asymptomatic individuals with normal electrocardiogram, the physician in charge should have a clear understanding of the pros and cons of a positive diagnosis in those who qualify for family screenings. The first aspect that should be considered is the potential harm that may derive from being identified as a silent carrier of a genetic defect. The second aspect that should be determined is the advantage provided by knowing that someone is a mutation carrier; this is predominantly defined by the nature of the disease and by the availability of measures (eg, lifestyle, medical treatments, diets) that a patient may adopt to reduce the risk of an adverse outcome or disease progression. The balance between the pros and cons of being identified as a mutation carrier determine for each family member whether genetic screening should be recommended.

Among factors that justify the screening of all family members, including those who are asymptomatic with normal QT interval, is the evidence that LQTS may cause life-threatening arrhythmias even in patients with a normal QTc,[3] especially in the presence of triggering environmental factors[4] such as the use of medications that prolong QT interval (www.qtdrugs.org), or the development of electrolyte abnormalities. The awareness of being a mutation carrier gives an individual the possibility of limiting exposure to factors that increase the arrhythmic risk, thus supporting the view that family members of an LQTS-genotyped individual benefit from genetic screening.

Another important aspect that supports the broad use of genetic testing among family members is provided by the use of prophylactic treatment with β-blockers to reduce the risk of arrhythmic events.[5]

For a family member without clinical signs of the disease, there are potential negative aspects of being tested. In some social settings, access to insurance coverage (health insurance and/or life insurance) may be denied to mutation carriers. In addition, social discrimination may be experienced by mutation carriers, including reduced chances of getting married or being hired. These factors should be weighed against the benefits and discussed with members of the family of a genotyped individual before genetic screening is recommended.

In our practice in Italy and the United States, we have found that most family members eventually decide that there is an advantage in being screened; if found to be mutation carriers, they can limit the exposure to arrhythmic triggers, carefully plan reproductive life, and, if considered appropriate by their physician, adopt prophylactic therapies. Because LQTS has an early onset and may also cause sudden death in the early years of life, family members of a genotyped proband are often screened during infancy and the prepuberal period.

CHALLENGES IN THE INTERPRETATION OF RESULTS OF GENETIC SCREENING IN LQTS

As soon as genetic testing became broadly available, it became clear that the challenge is not performing DNA screening but interpreting the results.

In North America, companies that provide genetic screening have introduced in their reports some clues to facilitate the interpretation of results. In Europe, research laboratories that provide a large proportion of genetic screening also provide results accompanied by some form of interpretation. Despite the support provided by these diagnostic laboratories, it is fundamental that results are critically interpreted by the clinical team in charge of the patient or by an external specialist before they are discussed with patients.

This article summarizes the approach that we use at our centers in Pavia and in New York to assess whether a DNA change is likely to cause LQTS.

The interpretation of the significance of a DNA variant is a complex task that requires time and caution before data are released. In our groups, the team interpreting complex mutations consists of a clinical geneticist, a molecular biologist, a cardiologist with training in channelopathies, and a basic scientist expert in cellular electrophysiology. Several approaches are combined to decide the meaning of DNA variants that are rare or of unclear significance.

The first step in interpreting a DNA change is to establish whether it has been found in normal individuals in the published literature, from open-source databases, or in our own control populations. As a second step, we determine whether the variant of interest has been reported in the medical literature in conjunction with the LQTS phenotype: these 2 steps can be accomplished by consulting online databases such as those listed in **Box 1**.

The next level of assessment of a DNA variant of unclear significance consists in retrieving from PubMed the published studies that have identified the variant to evaluate whether there is robust cosegregation between the DNA variant of interest and the clinical phenotype. We search to see whether any basic science experiment has been performed to characterize in vitro the functional consequence of the DNA variant.

Most of the genes that cause LQTS encode for proteins that form ion channels and therefore it is simple to perform investigations in heterologous systems (human embryonic kidney cells or Chinese hamster ovary cells) to test whether the channel engineered to carry the DNA variant of interest presents changes that alter the kinetics of the current or modify the localization of the protein to the cell membrane. Despite not knowing whether, when the protein is expressed in myocytes, it will present the same behavior that is seen in noncardiac cells, in vitro functional studies represent the most advanced way of testing

---

Box 1
Online genetic databases

http://www.ncbi.nlm.nih.gov/projects/SNP/

http://hapmap.ncbi.nlm.nih.gov/

http://ftp-trace.ncbi.nih.gov/1000genomes/ftp/

http://www.fsm.it/cardmoc/

http://www.genomed.org/LOVD/introduction.html

http://www.hgmd.cf.ac.uk/docs/oth_mut.html

whether a DNA VUS is able to alter the function of the encoded ion channel.

An additional approach that is adopted at our centers to predict the consequence of a mutation relies on the use of predictive software such as PolyPhen (http://genetics.bwh.harvard.edu/pph/) or SIFT (http://sift.jcvi.org/), which estimates the consequences of an amino acid substitution on the structure and function of the protein of interest.

Recently, in an attempt to help clinicians to interpret LQTS genetic testing, a large compendium of LQTS mutations was published.[6] This effort provides an exhaustive list of DNA variants identified in different laboratories around the world. However, the compendium provides little or no information about the phenotype present in the mutation carriers or the strength of cosegregation with clinical manifestations. It is therefore inappropriate to assume that a DNA change is pathogenetic simply because it is listed in a published compendium.

VUS: WHAT TO DO

Despite a substantial amount of time and effort invested in the interpretation of genetic results, it is still common that DNA variants identified in patients with LQTS cannot be properly classified; to reflect the uncertainty of their clinical meaning, these DNA changes are defined as VUS. VUS cannot be used in the clinical setting, because they are not informative enough to establish a diagnosis in patients with borderline QT interval or determine whether family members are affected by LQTS. Carriers of VUS are managed as if their genetic screening were negative (no mutation identified). Clinicians should be aware that, because of the constant improvement in knowledge of DNA variants in human genes, VUS will eventually be reclassified either as pathogenetic mutations or as polymorphisms and, therefore, physicians have to check with the laboratory that provided genetic testing on whether changes in the interpretation of a given VUS have occurred.

GENETIC COUNSELING: IMPORTANT TEAMWORK

Genetic counseling is a medical process intended to help patients and their families cope with the problems related to the diagnosis of a genetic disease. The successes obtained in genetic research and the increasing numbers of available genetic tests have made genetic counseling a fundamental part of the process of genetic evaluation. It is important to give patients all the information necessary to be autonomous in all their choices regarding the genetic diagnosis, the extension of the genetic diagnosis to healthy family members, and the therapeutic approaches suggested by the type of genetic mutation.

Genetic counseling should be performed by professionals with specific training who are prepared to give support to patients and their family members. In counseling families with LQTS, it is important to provide information on the clinical manifestations, prognostic implications, and inheritance patterns, as well as on the value of genetic screening and its implications.

Results of genetic testing should not be sent to the patients in the form of a written report; they should be given to the patients during a second consultation designed to explain the findings and their relevance for the index cases and their family members.

At our centers, genetic counseling is a multidisciplinary effort that consists of the 2 steps outlined in **Box 2**.

SUMMARY

This article provides an overview of the complexity of genetic testing in LQTS. Now that DNA screening for mutations in LQTS-related genes

---

Box 2
Two-step approach to genetic counseling

1. Prescreening counseling: patients obtain all the information needed to decide whether they want to undergo the screening and be informed about the results. During this first consultation, an informed consent to accept molecular screening of LQTS genes is obtained. Patients are also asked to decide whether they consent to have their DNA stored for future screening of new disease-related genes.

2. Postscreening counseling: the patient is informed of the results of the genetic testing and can decide, with the help of the cardiologist and the genetic counselor, about:

   a. The most suitable therapeutic approach, based on the information derived from the genetic testing.

   b. Screening of children younger than legal age.

   c. Communication of results to family members.

   d. Family planning for future pregnancies, including options of preimplantation genotyping and/or prenatal genotyping or genotyping at birth.

has become available to most patients, there is a growing need for clinicians with the expertise required for making conservative and appropriate use of genetic testing, recommending extension to screening to family members only when a clear benefit can be provided, and interpreting the results from the molecular laboratory. Interpreting the results requires the ability to collect information from different sources to define whether a DNA variant can be considered the cause of the disease. To provide patients with inherited arrhythmogenic diseases with a good standard of care, it is important to create a new subspecialty in clinical electrophysiology to train individuals with the expertise required to manage patients with these conditions.

REFERENCES

1. Bai R, Napolitano C, Bloise R, et al. Yield of genetic screening in cardiac channelopathies. Circ Arrhythm Electrophysiol 2009;2:6–15.

2. Ackerman MJ, Priori SG, Willems S, et al. HRS/EHRA expert consensus statement on the state of genetic testing for the channelopathies and cardiomyopathies: this document was developed as a partnership between the Heart Rhythm Society (HRS) and the European Heart Rhythm Association (EHRA). Heart Rhythm 2011;8:1308–39.

3. Priori SG, Schwartz PJ, Napolitano C, et al. Risk stratification in the long-QT syndrome. N Engl J Med 2003; 348(19):1866–74.

4. Yang P, Kanki H, Drolet B, et al. Allelic variants in long-QT disease genes in patients with drug-associated torsades de pointes. Circulation 2002; 105:1943–8.

5. Moss AJ, Zareba W, Hall WJ, et al. Effectiveness and limitations of beta-blocker therapy in congenital long-QT syndrome. Circulation 2000;101:616–23.

6. Kapplinger JD, Tester DJ, Salisbury BA, et al. Spectrum and prevalence of mutations from the first 2,500 consecutive unrelated patients referred for the FAMILION long QT syndrome genetic test. Heart Rhythm 2009;6:1297–303.

Index

Note: Page numbers of article titles are in **boldface** type.

Card Electrophysiol Clin 4 (2012) 103–105
doi:10.1016/S1877-9182(12)00018-4
1877-9182/12/$ – see front matter © 2012 Elsevier Inc. All rights reserved.

cardiacEP.theclinics.com

Moving?

Make sure your subscription moves with you!

To notify us of your new address, find your **Clinics Account Number** (located on your mailing label above your name), and contact customer service at:

Email: journalscustomerservice-usa@elsevier.com

800-654-2452 (subscribers in the U.S. & Canada)
314-447-8871 (subscribers outside of the U.S. & Canada)

Fax number: 314-447-8029

Elsevier Health Sciences Division
Subscription Customer Service
3251 Riverport Lane
Maryland Heights, MO 63043

*To ensure uninterrupted delivery of your subscription, please notify us at least 4 weeks in advance of move.

Printed and bound by CPI Group (UK) Ltd, Croydon, CR0 4YY

03/10/2024

01040351-0005